Dissolving Pain

Also by Dr. Les Fehmi and Jim Robbins

The Open-Focus Brain

Dissolving Pain

Simple Brain-Training Exercises
for Overcoming Chronic Pain

Les Fehmi, PhD, and Jim Robbins

 TRUMPETER · *Boston & London* · 2010

NOTE TO THE READER: This book is not intended as a substitute for medical advice or treatment.

TRUMPETER BOOKS
An imprint of Shambhala Publications, Inc.
Horticultural Hall
300 Massachusetts Avenue
Boston, Massachusetts 02115
www.shambhala.com

9 8 7 6 5 4 3 2 1

First Edition
Printed in the United States of America

⊗ This edition is printed on acid-free paper that meets the
American National Standards Institute Z39.48 Standard.
♻ This book was printed on 30% postconsumer recycled paper.
For more information please visit www.shambhala.com.

Distributed in the United States by Random House, Inc.,
and in Canada by Random House of Canada Ltd

Designed by James D. Skatges

Library of Congress Cataloging-in-Publication Data
Fehmi, Les.
Dissolving pain: simple brain-training exercises for overcoming chronic pain /
Les Fehmi and Jim Robbins.—1st ed.
p. cm.
Includes index.
ISBN 978-1-59030-780-9 (pbk.: alk. paper)
1. Chronic pain—Exercise therapy. 2. Alpha rhythm. 3. Visual evoked response. I.
Robbins, Jim. II. Title.
RB127.F44 2010
616'.0472—dc22
2010015975

Contents

Contents

Acknowledgments

I would like to herald the literary contributions of my coauthor Jim Robbins. He is a wordsmith of the highest order, who has deftly researched the context of the Dissolving Pain process. He was able to convert academic concepts into cogent prose, describing the subtle realities mentioned in this book. Without him, this enterprise could not have been executed or otherwise conceived.

I am pleased to acknowledge the many clients and staff whose efforts and practice contributed to the making of this book. My many thanks go especially to Phyllis Loften, Caroline Loften, and Bruce Ehmer, who tirelessly and energetically read and reviewed this book, typing its many revisions and catching important mistakes.

My thanks go to the staff of Shambhala Publications for their insight and valuable suggestions. Thanks to Ben Gleason and especially to Eden Steinberg, who is a gift to the literary arts and an insightful leader in accomplishing our goals.

I am grateful to my children, Laura, Jeff, and Emy Fehmi, who read and made many valuable suggestions.

The greatest personal and professional credit belongs to Susan Shor Fehmi who has worked with me in Open Focus, side by side, at the Princeton Biofeedback Centre for over thirty years. These are the wonderful years.

Dissolving Pain

Introduction

Renee is a lawyer who had her right knee joint replaced with an artificial one. In her hospital room the first night after surgery, her knee throbbed painfully, to the point that she could no longer bear it. The doctor had prescribed OxyContin, a powerful opiate for pain relief, but after she took it, her knee still throbbed. Moreover, the medication nauseated her and she couldn't sleep.

Renee, however, was prepared. Years earlier she had suffered from chronic lower back pain, and she had learned a powerful technique at our clinic for alleviating pain. I am a clinical psychologist and researcher, and for more than forty years, I've been teaching individuals how to improve their emotional and physical health using mental exercises in an approach I call Open Focus™. These exercises involve nothing more than changing the way we deploy our attention.

In the hospital that night, Renee took out a compact disc player and listened to an Open-Focus exercise that guided her in dissolving her physical pain. A few minutes after she began the exercise, the pain in her throbbing knee started to subside. Twenty minutes later, before the exercise was over, the pain was gone. She then used the exercise to help with the feelings of nausea. Within fifteen minutes, her stomach settled and she was able to sleep through the night.

Renee's story may sound remarkable, and yet at our clinic we hear many such stories from our patients. This book presents the techniques that Renee and others have used to alleviate pain of all kinds. It also explores recent scientific research demonstrating that pain, whatever its causes, resides principally in the brain and can therefore be treated by working with the mind in specific ways.

Martin's problem was different from Renee's. He suffered cluster headaches for years, and they greatly impacted the quality of his work in a demanding job as a stock trader in Manhattan. At first he worked through his headaches, trying to ignore the pain or taking ibuprofen for some relief. Cluster headaches—which can be so excruciatingly painful they are dubbed "suicide headaches"— are characterized by a sudden onset of sharp pain, usually on one side of the head, which last from fifteen minutes to several hours. They come in groups over a week or two and then subside for a while. When Martin's headaches worsened, he started taking prescription medication so that he could keep working. Finally, even with medication, the pain became unbearable.

He came to our clinic for help, and as he and I were talking, he said he could feel the faint beginnings of a headache (something sufferers call shadows). I took him into a treatment room, where he listened to exercises similar to those Renee had used. Then and there, his shadow headache went away and did not develop into a full-blown cluster headache that day.

Relief for both Martin and Renee came from following spoken-word exercises such as the ones you will find in this book, which guided them to pay attention to their physical pain in ways they don't normally do and allowed their bodies to quickly dissolve feelings of physical pain. The Open-Focus approach to pain consists of powerful yet simple techniques that are effective with almost any kind of pain, physical or emotional. And virtually anyone can learn them and use them to improve the quality of their lives.

We Have the Power to Heal Ourselves

The human central nervous system is the crowning achievement of nature, from the three-pound brain to the complex web of forty-five miles of nerves in our muscles and skin to our heart and stomach, which have smaller nervous systems of their own. This elegant biological equipment loves; creates art; reads books and watches movies; eats; enjoys nature and food; experiences feelings of fear, despair, transcendence, and, yes, pain. Yet we seldom think about the miracle that is our nervous system until a problem arises.

The nervous system is even more wondrous than we know. One of its greatest yet often unrecognized functions is the extent to which it is self-regulating. Many problems commonly seen as beyond our control, from anxiety to depression to physical pain, can be healed without prescribed medications or other medical interventions—if we know how. The control dial that engages this self-healing mechanism is how we pay attention—both to the world around us and to our inner world of thoughts and feelings.

Most of us are stuck in one mode of attention that I call narrow-objective focus. This is a highly concentrated, emergency mode of attending. It can be a productive and useful form of attention, allowing us to accomplish challenging tasks. But we tend to greatly overuse it, and, because it is our mind's emergency mode, it engages the high frequencies of the brain's electrical activities, keeping the nervous system in overdrive.

In my view, it is the overuse of narrow-focus attention that often leads to anxiety, depression, attention deficit disorder, muscle tension, and physical pain. When we discover the alternative styles of attention at our disposal and learn to use them, we can treat many problems on our own, including physical pain of almost any type. This book shows you how.

My wife and colleague, Susan Shor Fehmi, and I specialize in the treatment of pain, whether migraines, cluster headaches, neck and back pain, joint pain, phantom limb pain, pain from traumatic injury, or chronic pain anywhere in the body—as well as the emotional factors that often accompany and exacerbate physical pain, including anxiety and depression. We have effectively treated all these forms of pain simply by helping people change the way they deploy their attention. The techniques presented in this book are based on a series of experiments I conducted as a graduate student in the field of brain research. They are also based on our experience treating patients for the past thirty-five years at our clinic.

The take-home message of this book is that many kinds of chronic tension and pain, even tension we are unaware of or pain that seems entirely physical, can be eliminated or greatly eased by harnessing and using the different ways we are able to pay attention. The biggest mistake people in pain make is saying "Oh no, I've had migraines [or stomach pain or whatever] for years, and it's definitely physical. It really hurts, and it couldn't possibly be helped by my mind or how I pay attention." Mind and body function as one, however, and attention is the mechanism by which they are connected. Even the most physical of pain responds to how we attend.

I call the pain, tension, and other symptoms that are created by, or exacerbated by, how inflexibly we attend, *rigid attention syndrome*, or RAS. The solution is to undo the rigidity and become more flexible with our attention. It may be the most important thing we can do for our pain, for attention has power we simply don't recognize.

Pain is not something we must be stuck with. It is the product of operator error, an error we can learn to correct. Think of this book as an operator's manual that allows the human central nervous system to heal itself. You have far more control than you know.

How Are You Paying Attention?

How do you pay attention to your pain? This question may sound odd at first, but the fact is that we are paying attention to many things, including our pain, all the time whether we know it or not. The idea that we have choices about how we pay attention to pain—or that we have attentional choices at all—is a new concept to most and can initially seem confusing. But it is an old and simple concept that many cultures once knew about. It is a technique still used by some schools of meditation, though it is something Westerners have largely missed.

This book will introduce you to the different styles of attention available to us. It also features Open-Focus exercises you can use right away to begin to shift the way you pay attention so that your pain or discomfort, whether mild or moderate—be it a migraine, tissue damage, back pain, an itch, or nausea—is either diminished or dissolved. Even if the source of your pain is difficult to pinpoint, there is an exercise to help you find its center in the body and dissolve it.

Open-Focus exercises can help alleviate new pain that may have been caused by an injury, pain that is chronic, or pain that has cropped up seemingly for no reason, and they make us more resilient in the face of pain. (Of course, new pain or sudden increases in the intensity of previously existing pain should first be evaluated by a qualified physician.)

Pain and stress take a toll on many other aspects of our physiological and emotional life, including exacerbating anxiety, depression, and attention deficit disorder. Open Focus can help diminish these problems as well. In fact, work to alleviate pain often heals many of the other problems that can accompany pain.

Take the case of Ralph, a psychotherapist who came to see us because his lower back kept going into spasm. His frequent back pain made it difficult for him to sit and listen to his patients. "My back was going out three or four times a month," he said. "But within six weeks of using the Open-Focus exercises, I had total relief from the pain and didn't have another incident." For Ralph, the benefits went beyond pain relief. "I found that I could use Open-Focus attention when I was listening to my clients, which not only relieved any pain but helped me to become more in tune with my patients and much more alive during the sessions."

Ralph also says that since learning Open Focus, he feels that he's not living "in his head" all the time. "I'm much more in touch with what's going on around me. I'm more aware of simple things, like the changing of the seasons, which adds richness to my life."

Brian had severe headaches and muscle tension, pain so intense he was hospitalized twice. He took medication for the pain, which caused serious side effects. He also self-medicated with illegal drugs. Several months of Open-Focus training turned his life around. "If you met me six months ago, you wouldn't recognize me," he said. He was now able to manage his pain without taking any drugs. "The anxiety and the pain are both gone," he said. "Before I learned Open Focus, I wanted to stay in a shell all the time. Now I'm out there talking to people."

Alice had spastic colon, a painful condition that causes bowel spasms and diarrhea, along with severe headaches. She had been to several doctors and had also tried hypnosis, meditation, and other approaches. After she learned Open Focus, not only did her symptoms become rare, but she didn't worry as much and found she was more patient. "It generally made my life a lot easier to live."

There's an old saying: "Pain is inevitable, suffering is optional." Embark now on a journey in which you'll learn about your options when you're in pain. You'll discover that through the simple act of attending, you can help make suffering a thing of the past.

1

The Power of Attention

Attention is the nerve of the whole psychological system.

—Dr. Edward Titchener,
pioneering attention researcher

There's a joke in which two young fish swim by an older fish, and the old guy says to the youngsters, "Mornin', boys. How's the water?" "Fine," they answer. After they pass the old fish, one young fish turns to the other and says, "What the heck is water?"

There is a similar phenomenon at work with attention. If I were to ask you how you are paying attention right now, you might ask, "What does that mean?" Though we use our attention all the time, we rarely think twice about it. We don't pay attention to how we pay attention as we go through life, but the act of attending is one of the most vital things we do. You are doing it right now, as you read these words. How we attend affects us every moment of every day, and it is something we should all know a lot more about.

Have you ever wondered why you might feel open and generous one minute and feel anxious and critical the next? Why a pain in your leg pounds one minute and feels as if it is gone the next? The biggest factor in these kinds of changes is a spontaneous, unconscious shift in your style of attention. Pain, moods, and emotions are changed by shifts in attention all the time, but we usually don't realize it.

Most critically, attention also has everything to do with pain, stress, and tension, and how we perceive them. In fact, the story about the fish could apply to stress as well. We are so deeply immersed in our stress as it insidiously accumulates throughout our lives that we don't realize how stressed we really are. Attention helps us feel that stress and release it.

I define attention as *formed and directed awareness*. If we sit in a chair and our mind is empty of thought, we are simply aware. If a person walks into the room and we turn to see who it is, we have reached toward him or her with our awareness—and that reach is accomplished by use of certain types of attention. It may be easy to understand that we reach out into the world around us with our attention but it is more difficult to understand that we can also reach toward things we carry internally, such as emotions, thoughts, memories, and our pain, physical and emotional.

But why is the manner in which we form and direct our awareness so vital? Because certain kinds of attention quickly cause a widespread change in our physiology, including the dissolution of physical and emotional stress. Many therapies or relaxation techniques, from massage to tai chi to listening to music, produce positive results that succeed, at least in part, because they bring about a shift in attention. Even watching a movie can make us feel better because it shifts our attention. Attention, I believe, is the primary and most powerful factor in all types of relaxation.

It's important to emphasize that it is not only *what* we attend to that is important. What is as critical—and sometimes more critical—is *how* we attend, *how* we form and direct our awareness toward the object of our attention. This is a new concept for many. Most books and articles about improving attention talk about only one type, focused attention, which I call narrow-objective attention. The fact that as a culture we are not aware of other types suggests the degree to which we are addicted to narrow-objective attention.

In our culture, we are not taught to use the full repertoire of types of attention—the different styles, each with different qualities and each suited to different kinds of tasks and functions—because we're not aware of them. Instead, we are culturally biased to stay locked in this single mode of paying attention. I have spent the last forty years researching different styles of attention and applying them therapeutically, especially for the treatment of pain.

My discovery of how we can quell pain by changing how we are paying attention began in the mid-1960s, when I was engaged in research at the UCLA Brain Research Institute and later as a post-doctoral fellow. At that time, I was researching visual perception in monkeys. I was exploring the question of how the brain processes a visual signal and learned that the neurons that govern vision are activated simultaneously, rather than sequentially, in response to a stimulus.

This research led to a key discovery: the way the brain communicates with itself is through the use of brain-wave synchrony. I also learned from my doctoral research that when the brain's electrical activity is synchronized in more than one area of the brain, the brain can better perform its task. And the more each area of the brain has neurons working together—a kind of local synchrony—the better they can carry out their tasks.

To further my research, I began looking for ways that I could teach human subjects to encourage more electrical synchrony in their brain. Research taking place at that time showed that people could learn to control the electrical activity of the brain, as shown on an EEG (an electroencephalogram, which produces a graphical representation of the brain's electrical activity), so I would be able to do the same, with the help of technology coming on the scene known as biofeedback.

Biofeedback simply means feeding back to the user a signal about the body. Even though the technique is very simple, it allows a subject to learn quickly how to make relevant physiological changes. By holding a thermometer in your hand, for example, you can quickly learn to raise your fingertip temperatures and increase blood flow to different regions of your body, something that is difficult to do without the temperature feedback device.

Neurofeedback is a type of biofeedback that is based on brain waves. When sensors are attached to the scalp, enabling subjects to view their own brain frequencies, they can quickly learn to move into a relaxed, alert state, associated with a specific frequency, and dwell there.

I decided to begin by trying to encourage synchronous brain waves myself. Commercial biofeedback instruments weren't available when I started in 1967, so I built my own using an oscilloscope and a pen-and-ink EEG. I attached a sensor on the back of my head, with a reference and ground sensor on the ears.

On an EEG, our brain waves generally appear within the range of 0.1 to 40 hertz. (A hertz is the number of cycles per second. The higher the hertz, the higher the brain-wave frequency.) The lowest range of brain-wave activity is called delta, from 1 to 4 hertz, and it occurs predominantly during sleep. Theta activity, from 4 to 7 hertz, is the frequency range between sleeping and wakefulness. Alpha, from 8 to 12 hertz, corresponds to a state of being alert but relaxed. Above that, beta activity governs most of our daily activities (and corresponds to narrow-objective focus). In my experiment, I was looking for a way to get myself into alpha, the 8- to 12-hertz range.

I tried several ways to encourage alpha waves and put myself in a restful, relaxed state that would produce synchronous alpha brain waves. But I just couldn't do it and gave up. To my astonishment, the second I gave up, my alpha waves increased in both amplitude and abundance. It was the letting go of effort that finally produced alpha synchrony.

Then, as I learned to increase my production of alpha over the next few days, some delightful changes took place. The tone of my muscles softened, and I found I walked with a new kind of fluidity. Anxiety and irritability evaporated. I felt centered and poised. My senses improved, and when I walked outside, I could deeply smell the fragrance of the spring flowers and hear the birds. My somewhat obsessive-compulsive style mellowed, and I taught complex graduate-level courses with a newfound ease. People around me, students and family, responded positively. Yet I didn't feel that I had lost my edge—in fact, my teaching and research came easier and more clearly than before. *Moreover, I noticed that any tension and pain that I had been holding on to dissolved, and arthritic pain in my joints disappeared.*

The most important effect that I experienced was a reduction in tension, heaviness, and stress. The greatest surprise to me was that I hadn't realized the stress was present until it went away. Why didn't I know about it? Why did tension accumulate? How much more was still present? To what degree could I trust my personal experience to gauge or assess this tension?

The improvements I experienced as a result of my experiment with alpha synchrony lasted for months, and I found that if my gains started to diminish, a little more training could bring them back.

This was, I felt strongly, the way life was meant to be. I was in the zone.

Other researchers at this time had discovered the power of alpha brain waves, notably Dr. Joe Kamiya at the Langley Porter Neuropsychiatric Institute in San Francisco. He was able to teach student subjects to go into alpha at will, and the more they did so, the more they experienced this refreshed, relaxed state.

There was another very important, though more subtle, change that I observed. After several hours of brain-wave training, I noticed that my attention was expanded. That is, I took in the world visually in a very different way. I took in scenes broadly without overfocusing on any one element. I might look at a harbor with many boats and docks, and the ocean and the sky. Instead of seeing one or two boats on the water and then turning my gaze to see the dock over there, I saw the whole scene, all of the boats and everything else at once, rather than looking from one object to the next. My awareness of the world and my sense of it were also much bigger. This was my first experience with Open-Focus attention, a component of which is something I call diffuse attention.

There were two take-home messages from my experience. Producing alpha, the most synchronous of waking brain waves, caused my attention to shift from a narrow beam to an open, diffuse one and expanded my awareness. Second, I also realized that I could increase my production of alpha when I was living my everyday life, not just seated and connected to biofeedback equipment, simply by changing the way I paid attention.

I looked back at the research of Hans Berger, who discovered the existence of the brain's electrical output, and who reported in the 1920s on the association between alpha brain waves and a state of relaxed attentiveness.

If I learned to pay attention in an Open Focus—in which I saw the whole of the harbor scene with all of its objects, rather than picking out just one or two, and then did the same with the other senses simultaneously—perhaps I could produce synchronous alpha brain waves. Not just any kind of synchrony, but one called phase synchrony, in which many more regions of the brain are working together. While high-frequency beta activity is like people chattering in a church before the service starts, more open styles of attention generate a synchronized, uniform lower frequency across the brain, the equivalent of the congregation's singing a hymn together.

Flexible attention—moving from a narrow focus to a diffuse focus and back again—and other shifts of attention are at the heart of what this book is about, and it leads to the dissolution of rigid attention syndrome (RAS). We are culturally biased to stay in a narrow-objective focus, which increases the frequency of our EEG, tenses muscles, and generally *makes us more sensitive to pain,* sometimes unbelievably sensitive to the point that pain may be present with nothing to cause it (witness phantom limb pain). However, by and large, we don't know how and when to utilize the other styles of attention.

Attentional flexibility, however, is something that animals know intuitively and use to great advantage. If you have a house cat, watch it sometime as it lies awake but resting and is tempted by a toy at the end of a string. At first, the cat seems heavy-lidded, even half asleep. It takes in the world broadly. As the toy on the string approaches, the cat narrows its gaze on this object; all else is pushed to the background of the cat's perception. The cat sees only the toy. The animal has moved from a diffuse and immersed, resting style of attention, in which it takes in the world in a broad way, to a single-pointed visual focus that causes the animal's arousal level to rise: muscles tense, and heart and respiratory rates increase, as it prepares for the possibility of catching the toy at the end of the string.

This narrow and sometimes single-pointed way of attending is called narrow-objective focus. We may not realize it, but this is how the vast majority of us pay attention most of the time, not just visually but with all of our senses, to both our internal and external worlds. It is the focusing on one or a few important things as foreground and relegating everything else to the background of awareness, or even at times disregarding the background entirely.

Four kinds of attention form the awareness that we direct toward sense objects and perceptions. They are broken into two functions: scope (narrow or diffuse) and absorption (objective or immersed) attention. (These terms will be explored in depth later.)

While we can pay attention with all of our senses, vision, which uses about a third of our brain, is by far the most dominant, and how we pay attention visually has the greatest impact on our physiology. *Narrow-objective focus is an emergency mode of paying attention that quickly and substantially increases the frequency of the brain's EEG and raises other aspects of physiological arousal, which in turn directly affects our perception, emotions, and behavior.* And, by tensing muscles, it also creates new pain or exacerbates existing pain. Inappropriate muscle tension is also important because it hampers performance and is often a precursor to pain.

Our style of attention is reflected in the brain's electrical rhythms, the EEG. When we choose an attention style, we change the brain's electrical properties, which has systemwide effects, from muscle tension to heart rate to respiratory rate to the flow of blood, neurotransmitters, and hormones.

Narrow-objective attention is good for many tasks, but it is also a way of attending that is physiologically and psychologically taxing because it supports the accumulation of stress and tension. It also takes a great deal of effort to perpetually maintain this tension, even though we usually aren't aware of it.

We are equipped with this narrow beam of attention to respond to urgent or important external situations. There's nothing inherently wrong with narrow-objective attention; in fact, one reason it is overused is precisely because it is so helpful and allows us, in the short run, to accomplish so much. What's wrong is our almost constant use of it and dependence on it, our addiction to this single form, which leads to RAS. In narrow focus, we gain speed of processing in exchange for neurophysiological stability.

In the externalized, object-oriented society in which we live, narrow-objective focus is the way most people operate—and it's never questioned. We adopt it because it pays off, at least in the short run. We are both rewarded and criticized based on our ability to focus upon, objectify, recall, and verbalize our thoughts and experiences. "Pay attention to the teacher," we're told. "Stop daydreaming."

We've all been instructed and criticized like this, even though we were, of course, paying attention, even if it was to something else, in our own way, or to our own thoughts and ideas. What your parents or teacher really meant was that you weren't paying narrow enough attention to them, or what they felt was important, excluding everything else.

We use narrow-objective attention to focus on and grasp the thousands of distinctions among almost every sense experience that we have. We use computers, watch television, read books and newspapers, drive cars and go to museums, read legal briefs, and assemble automobiles. Each of these activities requires constant attention to the finest of details, and we have a highly refined and discriminating attention system to do all these things. We do almost all of them in narrow-objective attention.

At the bottom of some of our attention problems, however, are our repressed emotions. Just as the house cat experiences physiological changes when playing or hunting, human beings respond to problems and threats (real or perceived) by heightening their arousal and narrowing their focus to deal with immediate challenges. From the time we are very young, we respond to fearful situations by narrowing our scope of attention and distancing ourselves from the world, objectifying it, so we can assess and respond. Then we reflexively repress the feelings of fear that occur in our body by staying in narrow focus. Mind and body think and feel together. The problem is that, unlike the cat, we don't know how to shift back into a diffuse-immersed form of attention to recover, to allow feelings of fear to be released in nonemergency modes of attention. Instead, we keep our muscles tense, to prevent the feelings from surfacing in both the mind and the body.

Almost everyone suffers from overuse of chronic narrow-objective attention to some degree, predominantly due to emotional stress. Much of this habit originates in infancy and childhood, when we are too inexperienced to understand the world. Then this habit stays with us, along with an accumulation of stress.

Instead of learning to release fear, tension, and pain, we develop the habit of distracting ourselves from them, to keep us from feeling the discomfort we carry. Well-meaning adults unwittingly train us to turn away from pain and narrow our focus on something else. A skinned knee and tears might elicit a "Don't cry, have a piece of candy" or "I'll put on your favorite video to make you feel better." This teaches us to repress the pain. But these fearful feelings that we hold on to and collect throughout life create a less stable nervous system.

We rarely take into account what I believe is the largest factor in the perception of pain, the condition of the receiver of the pain—the central nervous system. Our perception, memory, information processing, performance, physiology, and emotional well-being are all organized by, and subordinate to, how we are paying attention. Thus attention orchestrates the life cycle of pain.

In simple terms, the brain is responsible for perceiving and registering pain. If it has become unstable because of paying attention chronically in emergency mode, it does a poor job of processing pain signals and is much more reactive and hypersensitive, registering pain that might have no physical cause or exacerbating minor pain to make it seem much worse than it is.

Chronic narrow-objective focus, then, often creates a behavioral loop. Perhaps we bang a shin. We fight the pain by narrow-focusing away from it, which engages the sympathetic nervous system, which heightens arousal. In normal situations, the pain will dissipate. But in many cases, fighting the pain in narrow focus engages a fight-or-flight response, and the pain may take on a life of its own in the brain. If we fear the pain, it assumes an added emotional component. And with this stress, including tense muscles, the symptoms don't get a chance to diffuse.

To take another example, you might get punched in the eye and it hurts, but you narrow your focus, tensing the muscles around your eye and cheek, which causes blood flow to restrict, and so the injury is less likely to heal quickly. It's a cycle. The pain surfaces, we narrow our focus away from it, create more fight-or-flight stress, with increased muscle tension and nerve tension, which makes the pain worse and discourages healing.

We do all this because we fear the pain. It's human to fear pain and react the way we do. It seems counterintuitive not to avert our attention or fight the pain. Think, though, what we do with pleasant feelings. We don't stop them and try to hold them back; we allow them in because they are pleasant—and, lo and behold, they dissolve on their own. We open up when we meet someone we like and talk to him or her, or we enjoy a good movie or go to a birthday party. If someone pays us a compliment, we feel good for a few minutes, or perhaps much longer, and after a while the feeling dissolves and goes on its way. Although it takes some work because of their noxious content, the same can be done with unpleasant feelings.

In the state of chronic narrow focus, pain takes on an outsize role in another way. The restricted scope of our focus is so small that the pain seems like a bigger deal than it is. When you are narrow-focused on something, including pain, it represents 100 percent of your awareness. When you broaden your attention beyond the pain, the pain becomes a fraction of your total awareness, a less formidable object to face and melt into.

Moving out of narrow-objective focus allows us to bring the pain into a more conscious awareness but at the same time makes the pain less formidable. It allows us to localize the pain—that is, to feel precisely where it is in the body—which is the critical first step toward dissolving it.

In the following chapters we'll look at the conventional understanding of pain and see how that model has undergone revision to a new model, one that accounts for why Open Focus and flexible attention work so well. The problem is that while some researchers have changed the pain model, most medical treatment is still based on the old model.

In my research, I found that the fastest way to break the hold of narrow focus is to become aware of space—space between objects, space in your body, space outside and even into the sky. So this book is interspersed with "space-based" exercises that first teach you how to move out of narrow focus into a more synchronous alpha state, in which pain is not such a big deal. While we use neurofeedback equipment in our clinic to enhance the effect of the exercises, you can get similar results using the exercises alone. The exercises are powerful and are the first step toward ending or ameliorating even the most stubborn pains, the ones you may have thought you were doomed to live with.

Exercise

Reading This Book in Open Focus

Even as you read this book, you can try a short exercise that will show you how to attend differently in your everyday life and how simple it can be to admit an awareness of space into your daily routine. Without shifting your eyes from the page, gradually become aware of the space that is to the right and the left of the page. Let your peripheral vision widen at its own pace to take in that awareness. As you develop that awareness, enjoy it for a few seconds.

Now allow your visual background to come forward, to become as important as your visual foreground. In other words, the whole page, the edges of the book, the table and walls behind the book, can be made foreground simultaneously with the words you are reading. This, too, should be carried out effortlessly and naturally. It may seem difficult at first, but it is well within our capacity to focus this way. Sit for a few seconds as you gently maintain this awareness and allow background and foreground to become equally important or interesting.

As you continue reading, also include the space that surrounds your entire body. Allow time for the perception to take place as your visual awareness opens and broadens into three dimensions. Now permit yourself to become aware of the space between the lines you are reading, even as you continue to read. Also bring into your awareness the space between the words themselves, and then the space between the letters of the words. Your awareness of visual space can continue to expand effortlessly while your awareness of letters, words, and concepts continues.

Expanding your three-dimensional visual awareness of space is creating a change in the way you have habitually paid attention. You may also begin to sense your awareness expanding into other sensations of the absence we call space—feeling it, tasting it, smelling it, hearing silence, experiencing the space and silence in your mind from which visual and internal dialogue emerges, along with a limitless sense of now.

As you continue to allow your awareness to open and become more inclusive, you may notice subtle alterations in the experience of the material you are reading. Your understanding of the content might become more centered, enriched, and engaged. It may become easier to read the words. Thoughts of things unrelated to what you are reading might float effortlessly through your mind. Your eyes may feel less strained. The hand that supports the book may feel more relaxed. Breathing may come more easily. You may discover that tension or even minor pain in the muscles in your face and neck is dissolving or that your position in your chair has become more comfortable. You may feel more whole or unified. You may also sense some mildly unpleasant feelings rising up—feelings that have been repressed by the act of narrow focusing. Methods for dissolving these will be discussed in a later chapter.

If you notice even small changes during the reading exercises, you have begun to experience some of the benefits of becoming aware of space. It may seem strange, even uncomfortable at first, for we all have learned to pay narrow and effortful attention to what we read and to most other things. Narrow-objective focus is thought to be necessary to resist distractions so we can understand, analyze, and do something about what we read. That idea is so ingrained that many of us have become unaware of rigid attention syndrome (RAS), the mental and physical stress and fatigue, tension, and even pain that accompany this constant gripping. Our eyes grip the words, our mind grasps the concepts, our fingers may literally clutch the book.

But we don't need this level of effort merely for reading. Open Focus, on the other hand, releases this effortful attention and allows us to expend just the right amount of effort rather than chronically overdoing it. A precise, relaxed, yet interested attention—a lightly held narrow-objective attention amid a diffuse-immersed background of space—is maintained, while tension and stress and pain dissolve.

You can use this exercise while doing almost anything, from riding the subway to talking on the phone, cooking, or working on your computer. Stopping what you are doing and becoming aware of your peripheral vision, of the space between you and the objects around you, is a way to begin incorporating Open Focus into everyday life.

2

A New Approach to Pain

Pain is a more terrible lord of mankind than death itself.
—Albert Schweitzer

In my previous book, *The Open-Focus Brain,* I described an important moment early on in my career that created for me a new way of thinking about pain. One day at work, I was seized by a sharp, sudden pain in my lower back caused by a kidney stone. (This was a reoccurrence of earlier episodes of excruciating kidney-stone pain. Remember to seek prompt medical attention if you experience severe pain of unknown origin.) It was the worst pain I have ever felt, a shuddering, all-encompassing pain. It was all I could do to remain standing long enough to find a chair. Pain medications did nothing. Neither did creating a competing pain, such as bending back a finger or pinching myself.

That evening, though, the pain went away completely, as suddenly as it began.

The next day, the pain returned. In an act of desperation I decided to try something different, something that seemed counterintuitive. Instead of reflexively fighting the pain, I surrendered to it. I stopped tensing muscles, and I allowed myself not only to fully feel the pain but to let it in and accept it, to merge with it. Almost immediately the pain ceased, and the world around me grew brighter and the pain was replaced by a feeling of lightness. I realized that a *major factor in how I experienced the pain was how I paid attention to it.* Instead of fighting the pain by narrowing my awareness onto it, resisting it, and avoiding it, I had broadened my awareness by opening to all my senses, and to space, putting the feeling of kidney pain squarely in the center of this expanded awareness. *When I attended that way, the pain became a small part of my total awareness, and with the pain now a small part of my being, I could easily surrender into the pain and dissolve it.*

To my astonishment, the pain was gone for a full day.

The next day, the pain returned, and the wonderful brightness I had experienced disappeared as the pain throbbed. I repeated the experience from the previous day and dove back into the pain. And again, the feeling of brightness and clarity came over me as the pain immediately dissolved. Again, any sudden, severe pain should be first attended to by a doctor, but I saw that we can do a lot to help ourselves to manage pain.

You might ask, "How can you dissolve pain simply by changing the way you pay attention?" The answer lies in the brain. The brain is the master control center that governs the nervous system, which in turn governs muscle tension, heart rate, and many other aspects of our physiology. While the severity of tissue damage or structural deficiencies is obviously important, the brain is where the pain experience is generated and where we can intervene in the pain network. And we intervene by changing how we pay attention.

Nothing illustrates this better than the phenomenon of phantom limb pain, pain that persists in a limb after it has been removed. Take the example of Rob, a client who came into my Princeton Biofeedback Centre on crutches. A traffic accident years ago had damaged his right leg, and it had been amputated near the top of the thigh. Lately, however, he told me he had started to suffer severe knee pain in his amputated right leg, which ached at night and kept him from sleeping. He felt a little sheepish admitting this to me; his leg was gone, for crying out loud. How could his knee hurt?

Rob's complaint has been a conundrum in the world of pain for a long time. Some 95 percent of amputees have such pain, and it can last throughout their lives, according to the medical literature. The scientific record goes back to the Civil War and to a doctor of that era named Silas Weir Mitchell, who amputated a large number of infected and injured limbs (as was the standard treatment of the time). Amputees complained to him that they felt haunted by their vanished limbs. Dr. Mitchell described his patients' perceptions as a "sensory ghost" and later coined the term *phantom limb*. In addition to feeling pain in a missing limb, people sometimes see their missing arm or hand waving or reaching for things. Some leg amputees say they experience sensations in their missing feet and legs during sex. Other amputees say they continue to reexperience the moment of injury again and again.

During Rob's first treatment session at our clinic, we connected him to our neurofeedback equipment. Neurofeedback, or EEG biofeedback, took off in the 1970s after Joe Kamiya announced in *Psychology Today* his discovery that people could be taught to control their brain waves. Others soon were able to achieve the same kind of results. A number of researchers and manufacturers rushed to develop equipment that would give subjects the ability to move into stress-reducing alpha brain-wave patterns. But the hype got ahead of the science, and criticism, some fair and some not, caused the field to collapse and nearly disappear. Research funds dried up as some researchers and manufacturers of biofeedback equipment made unsupported claims that neurofeedback was a shortcut to feelings of transcendence. It was unfortunate, for there was a very real scientific phenomenon to be explored. Still, a few people persisted with further development of the technology, myself included, and got good results.

For example, Dr. Maurice "Barry" Sterman, a researcher at Sepulveda Veterans Hospital and a professor at UCLA, used neurofeedback in the 1970s to teach lab animals and then humans to control epileptic seizures. The results were significant. In one published study, he reduced the number of seizures in patients with severe epilepsy—so severe, drugs couldn't control the seizures, and they were waiting for radical surgery—by 60 percent. In another study published in the journal *Epilepsia,* he was able to train subjects not only to greatly reduce or eliminate their seizures but also to then increase their seizures in order to prove the methodology.

Since the mid-1990s, neurofeedback has made a comeback, with the help of sophisticated computer equipment that has made the technique much more powerful. There are now hundreds—possibly thousands—of practitioners around the world using neurofeedback techniques to help their clients alleviate a wide range of health problems.

New research on neurofeedback is promising. A 2010 paper published in the *European Journal of Neuroscience* confirmed that under rigorous laboratory conditions subjects could learn to control their brain waves, which made "a lasting change in cortical excitability." In other words, subjects were able to calm and regulate the electrical activity in their brains in an ongoing way. The authors called neurofeedback "a promising tool to modulate cerebral plasticity [to change the brain] in a safe, painless, and natural way."

There are many different types of neurofeedback, many different theories and treatment protocols. My own approach uses five channels, or five sites, on the scalp where I place small sensors to pick up the brain's electrical activity at each of the sites. When all five of these sites move into alpha (around 10 hertz), the machinery that is attached to the sensors gives the client "feedback" in the form of a light flashing and a beep sounding. Our clients are instructed to let the light and the beep activate as much as possible. This process encourages the brain to go into phase-synchronous alpha, with all five parts of the brain producing in-phase activity.

At first it's not easy for clients to let the light go on and the beep sound, so while they are attached to the neurofeedback equipment, we have them listen to Open-Focus exercises that ask them to become aware of space. Listening to the exercises helps them to move more quickly into phase-synchronous alpha, where they get a sense of what life outside of narrow-objective focus feels like. As Rob sat in a chair, he was asked to become aware of the space around him, behind, above, and below, which broadened his sense of awareness. I asked him, as I asked all my clients, to remain open to, and become broadly immersed in, all of the senses and to the space experienced in and through the periphery of attention.

Once he was in Open Focus, I led him through a Dissolving Pain exercise. After fifteen minutes, I asked him to imagine moving toward his pain, to stop fighting the pain, which was now much smaller and less intense in this expanded awareness, and to melt into it as I had with my kidney pain. Within half an hour, the pain he had when he came in that day had subsided. With regular practice, Rob learned he could completely dissolve his pain by frequently adopting alternative styles of attention, just as many hundreds of my other clients, with dozens of different kinds of pain, have been able to do.

Numerous hypotheses have been proposed to explain phantom limb pain. Some suggest there are active nerve endings at the point where the limb was severed, but the pain occurs even in patients whose wounds are well healed. And the pain sometimes occurs in other parts of the limb—a long way from where the limb was severed.

The reason the pain is still felt in the missing limb is because it is generated by the neurons in the brain that govern that part of the body. According to a chapter about phantom limb expert V. S. Ramachandran in Dr. Norman Doidge's book *The Brain That Changes Itself,* "Our pain maps get damaged and fire incessant false alarms, making us believe the problem is in our body when it is in our brain. Long after the body has healed, the pain system is still firing and the acute pain has developed an afterlife."

But the pain-generating neurons in the brain can be changed. Research in the 1990s—the so-called decade of the brain because of the commitment of funding to neuroscience—led to the key finding that the brain and nervous system are surprisingly plastic, or malleable. And my own work shows that we engage that plasticity and change the EEG frequency of those pain-creating neurons by changing how we pay attention, even if we don't realize how we are paying attention to pain or that we are paying attention to it at all.

This and other ideas about attention led to a career in which I have learned one important lesson: appropriately deploying attention is the sine qua non for mental, emotional, and physical health. When we learn to use our attention skills flexibly, in a way that is appropriate for each situation, we gain the power to profoundly change the way we relate to our world on every level—physically, emotionally, and mentally. Most important, we gain power over pain by changing how we pay attention. Open-Focus attention changes the frequency of neuronal activity, which alters the experience of pain.

Pain can be crippling and all-consuming—it separates us from our loved ones and our surroundings, condemning us to a private, isolating world of suffering. If it is chronic—that is, if it lasts beyond the time it usually takes to physically heal—it can drain the joy from life. Pain can keep us from doing our best at our job. Chronic pain can take us out of our robust three-dimensional world, where we are happy and enjoy life to the fullest, and confine us to a flat, two-dimensional one, where we are physically and emotionally drained due to the constant battle with pain. Pain can bring on depression and anxiety.

But pain is not necessarily a bad thing. Like stress, pain is an alarm that signals the need to attend to it and then to begin a response to end the painful experience. If you touch a hot stove, the pain tells you to withdraw. Pain, however, often lasts too long, is more severe than it should be, or takes on a life of its own. That's a signal there's something amiss, perhaps in the tissue, but also in the central nervous system.

Pain has many different definitions; in this book, I broadly refer to pain as any unwanted physical sensation, from a toothache to a migraine to an itch to nausea to deep, throbbing pain in muscles, tendons, or ligaments or a sharp, well-defined pain. Some pain is localized; some is all over and vague. It might be sharp, stabbing, burning, dull, fuzzy, shooting, pulsating, quivering, pounding, wrenching, cramping, or throbbing. Even emotional pains, such as anxiety and depression, are pains we can dissolve.

In the Open-Focus approach, all physical and emotional pain is treated in the same way.

Pain is highly subjective. The pain experience varies not only from person to person but from culture to culture. Two people can have completely different pain experiences in response to exactly the same wound. Genetics also plays a major role in pain perception. Redheads, for example, are as a rule more susceptible to some kinds of pain. A recent study in the *Journal of the American Dental Association* found that redheads are twice as likely as people with other hair colors to avoid going to the dentist because they are more susceptible to pain. And redheads also get less relief from pain medications.

Some seventy-five million Americans live in chronic pain, and one in three of those cannot maintain an independent lifestyle because of the pain, according to a national pain survey in 1999. Some 80 percent of the people who visit their doctor go for the treatment of pain of some kind, most often for back pain, which is second only to the common cold. People spend considerable sums seeking relief. The pain-management industry is expected to be worth more than $40 billion by 2011, according to Global Industry Analysts, a firm that tracks business statistics.

According to the World Congress on Pain, there is more than $80 billion a year lost in sick days and poor productivity, largely caused by headaches, back pain, and arthritis. Meanwhile, some of the commonly accepted solutions for pain—highly addictive medications such as codeine and morphine—cost society millions of dollars, and more when they are abused, and cause much more suffering in many who use them.

Of course, the tragedy is that very little of this pain treatment cures pain; it merely relieves it for a while, which is especially true of medication. The root cause often goes unaddressed. "We certainly cannot succeed as a culture," wrote David Morris in his book *The Culture of Pain,* "by continuing to deny and ignore pain, as if we could silence it beneath a mountain of pills."

Pain is obviously a major theme in our culture.

At the same time, experts say most pain is what is called somatoform pain. That means while the experience of body pain is real, it has no discernible cause. It likely resides in th brain. One recent survey, by Johannes Gutenberg University Mainz, in Germany, of 308 patients, found that 80 percent of the complaints to general practitioners were for somatoform pain.

Much of the suffering from chronic pain is unnecessary and has to do with how we pay attention and our too-limited awareness of space, something I will discuss in more detail later in the book. But for now try a short exercise that guides you through a sense of space and see how powerfully it changes your sense of awareness.

Exercise

A FEELING OF SPACE

General Introduction
to the Guided Exercises

Open-Focus exercises consist of a series of guiding questions that will help you to develop beneficial new styles of attention, which in turn will help you to alleviate pain. In these exercises, you will be asked to imagine certain experiences. Can you imagine letting your mind and body respond naturally to the questions without exerting any particular effort to achieve any one of these images or experiences?

For example, when I ask, "Can you imagine feeling the distance between your eyes?" you might naturally experience your eyes and then let your imagination flow to the region between your eyes and imagine feeling the space between them. Your objective is not to come up with some precise number or other abstraction, such as, "The distance between my eyes is two inches." The objective is to very gently imagine or experience that distance or region between your eyes. You might initially imagine or experience the distance as a very small region or vague feeling, and the distance might then expand or change as you continue to maintain your focus on that region. The experience often changes with continued practice. Opening your awareness to your emerging experience is a process that naturally shifts and changes over time.

As you proceed through the exercises, you'll notice that many of the questions involve imagining the space in and around your hands and fingers. Though this might seem a random part of the body to be focusing on, it is not. A larger portion of the brain is dedicated to controlling and sensing the hands and fingers than any other part of the body. So when we are attending to our hands and fingers in Open Focus, we're engaging a relatively large percentage of the brain—in other words, we're moving more of the brain into synchronous alpha.

Please allow approximately fifteen seconds between questions. For that period, I would like you to maintain your attention on the subject of the last question. If you have any difficulty imagining a particular image or experience, don't let that trouble you. Just permit your imagination to remain oriented toward the object of the question and let your experience evolve naturally. If nothing particular seems to happen or your mind wanders, don't be disturbed. In the event that you happen to notice that your attention has wandered and is focused upon some thought, image, or feeling, neither resist nor encourage this process. Merely allow your attentional focus to expand, to include also the image of the current Open-Focus question, in addition to the perception to which your mind has wandered.

Although most people find it helpful to close their eyes while doing the Open-Focus exercises, after some facility is gained, the practice may be done with eyes open or half open. Practicing with eyes fully or partially open enhances the transfer of the Open Focus to daily life. A relatively erect body posture is also recommended, either sitting or standing. Reclining positions are seldom effective, since they encourage sleep. Although drifting in and out of sleep may be a necessary developmental stage in the course of learning Open Focus, deep sleep and the associated loss of muscle tone are to be avoided.

Finally, you needn't respond overtly in any way to these questions. Your response will be whatever happens to your imagery or experience when the question is asked.

Audio Recordings of the Exercises

Though Open-Focus exercises appear in print in this book, for many people it's best to listen to them rather than read them. Audio recordings of two essential exercises for dissolving pain are included on the enclosed CD (attached to the inside back cover). For information on how you can download these recordings, please see page 183.

For the exercises that are not included on the audio CD, such as the one that follows, you can have someone read the guiding questions to you, or you can use a recording device to record them yourself. Either way, be sure to leave a fifteen-second pause after each question. (Recordings of all the exercises in this book are available for purchase at www.openfocus.com.)

Finally, the appendix explains how you can structure the exercises of the book into an ongoing, personal program for dissolving pain.

About This Exercise

This Open-Focus exercise, "A Feeling of Space," is intended to acquaint the reader with a subtle experience of space. Developing an awareness of space is key to learning to dissolve pain.

Remember to allow fifteen seconds between the end of one question and the beginning of the next question.

Guiding Questions

Can you imagine paying attention to the feeling of space that the whole room occupies?

Can you imagine paying attention to the feeling of space that your whole body occupies?

Can you imagine feeling the sense of presence of your thumbs?

Can you imagine paying attention to the feeling of space that your thumbs occupy?

Can you imagine paying attention to the feeling of space around the sense of presence of your thumbs?

Can you imagine paying attention to the feeling that the boundaries of your thumbs are dissolving?

Can you imagine paying attention to the feeling that the space inside your thumbs is continuous with the space outside your thumbs?

Can you imagine feeling the sense of presence of your index fingers?

Can you imagine paying attention to the feeling of space around the sense of presence of your index fingers?

Can you imagine paying attention to the feeling that the boundaries of your index fingers are dissolving?

Can you imagine paying attention to the feeling that the space inside your index fingers is continuous with the space outside your index fingers?

Can you imagine paying attention to the feeling of space between the thumb and index fingers on each hand?

In slow motion, can you imagine paying attention to the moving of your thumbs and index fingers toward each other and alternately away from each other, while attending to the feeling of the space between them, increasing and decreasing, narrowing and widening?

Can you imagine the feeling of space between your thumbs and index fingers on each hand (a space known as the purlicue) as a model for the feeling of space elsewhere in your body?

Can you imagine paying attention to the feeling of space between all of your fingers, just as you feel the purlicue between your thumb and index finger?

Can you imagine paying attention to the feeling of space that all your fingers occupy and the space around all your fingers, just as you feel the purlicue between your thumbs and index fingers?

Can you imagine paying attention to the feeling of space between the object of your attention and you, the observer?

Can you imagine paying attention to the feeling of space between your eyes?

Can you imagine paying attention to the feeling of space between this printed page, upon which the words and letters appear, and you, the observer?

Can you imagine paying attention to the feeling of space between you, the observer, and the words on the printed page?

Can you imagine paying attention to the feeling of space between you and the letters and words on the printed page?

Can you imagine that with practice you could continue to read while remaining attentive to all of the above spaces simultaneously?

Can you imagine what it would feel like if you were already successful at reading while remaining attentive to all of the above spaces simultaneously?

3

The Conventional
Understanding of Pain

To understand the Open-Focus model of pain, which is in keeping with other emotion-based models, it helps to have an understanding of the old model of pain—which, unfortunately, still governs most treatment.

The word *pain* is derived from Roman mythology: *Poena* is the Roman spirit of punishment, who serves Nemesis, the goddess of divine retribution. The Greek goddess of revenge was named *Poine*, sent when the gods were angry. For centuries, pain was seen as suffering inflicted by the gods, and many early treatments for pain consisted of magic and rituals to appease them. In Judeo-Christian thought, pain has also been understood as a punishment from God, as in the case of Job, whom God tested by inflicting physical and emotional pain.

Some Greeks and Romans, however, advanced a different notion: that the brain and nervous system had a role in producing the perception of pain. Zeno, for example, considered pain a form of grief. Later, during the Renaissance, the artist and expert anatomist Leonardo da Vinci posited that the brain was the central organ responsible for the sensation of pain. He also hypothesized that the spinal cord was a conduit that carried pain signals to the brain.

In the seventeenth and eighteenth centuries, there were numerous new hypotheses about the workings of the body, and the pain model evolved. In 1640, the French philosopher René Descartes described what he called a *pain pathway*, a term still used today. In an illustration, Descartes showed how fire, in contact with the foot, sent a signal that traveled up the leg and the body to the brain, where it "rang a bell," causing the sensation of burning pain.

Known as the *specificity* model, Descartes's centuries-old idea is still the most widely known and accepted theory of pain: if we prick our finger with a needle, there's damage to the tissue, which causes pain to travel along nerve fibers to the brain and ring the pain bell. In this model, the amount of pain we feel is the result of the type of injury and the severity of the injury to the body (and for this reason it is called the specificity model). A knife cut is more painful than a needle prick, for example. In the twentieth century, this model was still ascendant, and so the focus of much pain research was to discover the specific pain-conducting nerve fibers in the body.

Despite abundant research suggesting that the specificity model is woefully inadequate, modern medical practitioners still largely view pain this way—they focus exclusively on locating and repairing an injury to the body, with the understanding that this injury is sending out the pain signal, and so this is where the pain must be stopped. Much of modern surgery is based on this idea, often completely ignoring the lesson about the role of the brain in pain that comes to us from the phenomenon of phantom limbs.

A short history of the management of pain during surgery offers insight into where pain originates. Back in the old days, before anesthesia, a good doctor was one who could work fast and get the operation finished quickly to minimize pain. The first solution to alleviating the pain of surgery was invented by Franz

Anton Mesmer, a German physician who developed what he called animal magnetism, an early form of hypnosis. Mesmerists traveled Europe demonstrating the dramatic pain prevention of their craft, showing that people in a trance could have a pistol shot off next to their ear or their skin pricked or receive electric shocks and not feel it.

That led to the use of mesmerism, or hypnosis, for surgery. The first patient on whom the technique was used was a laborer who underwent several days of hypnotic induction to have his leg amputated. He exhibited no signs of pain, except for a low moaning that continued throughout the operation, which didn't seem related to the pain and never changed, even as the surgeon sawed through nerves. Afterward the patient said he felt no pain.

Hypnosis, in which attention plays a key role, was one of the first challengers to the specificity model—though today its lesson is largely ignored. A hypnotic state is one in which the person's attention becomes absorbed in relaxing thoughts and feelings and distracted from painful ones, and it clearly shows that there is more going on than a signal being transmitted from the site of the pain to the brain.

The use of hypnosis in treating pain is well studied and well documented. In a review of eighteen published studies, researchers writing in the *International Journal of Clinical and Experimental Hypnosis* found that those who underwent hypnosis as part of surgery reported significantly less pain and had a faster recovery. In a study published in the same journal, of 241 patients who underwent surgery, those who received self-hypnosis instructions had much less pain and anxiety than those who had no instruction. Research "substantiates the claim that hypnotic procedures can ameliorate many psychological and medical conditions," wrote authors of another study, in 2004, published in the journal *Anesthesia and Analgesia*.

It's long been observed that emotions can play a dramatic role in the perception of pain. One of the often-cited examples took place during World War II and was described by Dr. Henry K. Beecher, a medical officer admitting casualties to an army hospital (and later an expert in pain at Harvard). Beecher made a remarkable observation about the soldiers wounded on the battlefield at Anzio, where serious injuries were numerous. When admitted to the field hospital, these soldiers were asked if they were in pain and if they needed pain medication (morphine). A remarkable 70 percent said that they weren't in pain and didn't need morphine.

When he returned to the States, Beecher conducted a test with civilians who had similar injuries. He asked each person the same two questions he had asked the soldiers wounded at Anzio: are you in pain, and do you want morphine? This time, 70 percent said yes to both questions. He hypothesized that the difference in the perception of pain was caused by the fact that the wounds meant very different things to the two groups. The soldiers he treated were largely relieved, almost ecstatic: they had survived the battle and the wound meant they were getting away from the battlefield, away from the war, and possibly being sent home. The injured civilians, however, faced major disruptions to their lives as the result of their wounds, such as serious difficulties functioning and the loss of income. Beecher's observations, about how these two groups perceived the pain from similar injuries differently, was a first step toward a new model of pain that looked beyond the severity of the wound to the emotional state of the injured person.

The phenomenon of pain is clearly far more complex than Descartes ever imagined. As the *Oxford Companion to the Mind* puts it, "Pain is a complex perceptual and affective experience determined by the unique past history of the individual, by the meaning to him of the injurious agent or situation, and by his state of mind at the moment, as well as by the sensory nerve patterns evoked by physical stimulation."

Despite these revelations, most medical professionals still adhere to Descartes's model. In the last few decades, however, researchers have turned away from the notion of specificity to study a more complex model, one that includes the condition of the central nervous system and emotional stress. That's very much in keeping with the Open-Focus model, which asserts that the preponderance of the pain experience is governed not by the injury but by the brain and attention.

Exercise

Head and Hands

The purpose of this exercise is to develop your awareness of physical space in preparation for using the Open Focus exercises to dissolve pain. This exercise invites you to experience the space in and around your head, neck, shoulders, and hands in greater detail and depth.

Why spend time imagining space? Remember that when we shift our attention toward an awareness of space, this creates beneficial changes in the brain's electrical rhythms, which in turn lead to reduced stress and enhanced well-being.

As with all the exercises in this book, be sure to allow fifteen seconds between the guiding questions, and for that period maintain your attention on the subject of the last question. If you have difficulty imagining any particular image or experience, don't let that trouble you. Just permit your imagination to remain oriented toward the question and let your experience evolve naturally.

Guiding Questions

Can you imagine letting your mind and body naturally and effortlessly respond to the following questions about your ability to imagine certain experiences?

Can you imagine not giving any particular effort to listening to the questions or to achieving any of the associated images or experiences?

Can you imagine that the ideal response is whatever spontaneously happens to your imagery or experience when a particular question is asked?

Can you imagine that your opening and expanding awareness of your experience is a continuing process?

Can you imagine the distance between your eyes?

Is it possible for you to imagine the space inside your nose as you inhale and exhale naturally?

Can you imagine your breath flowing behind your eyes as you inhale naturally?

Can you imagine the distance between the space inside your nose and your eyes?

Can you imagine the space inside your throat as you inhale naturally?

Is it possible for you to imagine the distance between the space inside your throat and the space inside your nose?

Can you imagine the space inside your mouth and cheeks?

Is it possible for you to imagine the surface of your tongue?

Is it possible for you to imagine the entire region contained within the surface of your tongue; that is, can you imagine the volume of your tongue?

Can you imagine the volume of your teeth and gums?

Can you imagine the volume of your lips?

Is it possible for you to imagine the distance between your upper lip and the base of your nose?

Can you imagine the distance between the space inside your throat and the tip of your chin?

Can you imagine the space inside your ears?

Is it possible for you to imagine the distance between the space inside your throat and the space inside your ears?

Can you imagine the distance between the tip of your chin and the space inside your ears?

Can you imagine the distance between your ears?

Can you imagine the distance between the tip of your chin and your temples?

Can you imagine the distance between your temples?

Can you imagine the distance between the tip of your chin and the top of your head?

Can you imagine the distance between the tip of your chin and the back of your neck?

Can you imagine the distance between the tip of your chin and your cheekbones?

Can you imagine the distance between your cheekbones?

Is it possible for you to imagine the distance between the tip of your chin and your eyes?

Can you imagine the distance between your eyes?

Can you imagine the distance between the tip of your chin and the middle of your forehead?

Can you imagine the distance between the tip of your chin and the corners of your mouth?

Can you imagine the distance between the tip of your chin and your lower lip?

Can you imagine the distance between the corners of your mouth and your nostrils?

Is it possible for you to imagine the volume of your entire jaw?

Can you imagine the distance between your nostrils?

Can you imagine the space inside the bridge of your nose?

Can you imagine the distance between the space inside the bridge of your nose and the back of your head?

Can you imagine the distance between the space inside the bridge of your nose and your eyes?

Is it possible for you to imagine that the region around your eyes is filled with space?

Can you imagine the volume of your eyelids?

Can you imagine the distance between your eyelids and your eyebrows?

Is it possible for you to imagine the volume of your forehead?

Can you imagine the distance between the space inside the bridge of your nose and a point in the middle of your forehead?

Can you imagine the distance between the space inside the bridge of your nose and your hairline?

Is it possible for you to imagine the volume of your entire face simultaneously, including your ears, your jaw, your nose, and your tongue, your teeth, your gums, and your lips?

Can you imagine at the same time the volume of your scalp?

Can you imagine that as you inhale naturally your breath fills the entire volume of your face, scalp, and head, including your ears, jaw, and eyes?

Can you imagine that as you exhale and as your breath leaves your body it leaves your face, scalp, and head empty, that is, filled with space?

Can you imagine the space inside your throat expanding until your entire neck is filled with space?

Can you imagine the distance between the space inside your neck and the tips of your shoulders?

Can you imagine the space inside your throat and neck expanding to fill the entire region of your shoulders?

Can you imagine the volume of your upper arms?

Is it possible for you to imagine the volume of your upper and lower arms simultaneously?

Can you imagine the volume of your arms and your hands simultaneously?

Is it possible for you to imagine the volume of your thumbs?

Can you imagine the volume of your first fingers?

Is it possible for you to imagine the space between your thumb and first finger on each hand?

Can you imagine the volume of your middle finger on each hand?

Can you imagine the space between your first finger and your middle finger on each hand?

Is it possible for you to imagine the volume of your fourth finger on each hand?

Can you imagine the space between your middle and fourth fingers?

Can you imagine the volume of your little fingers?

Can you imagine the space between your fourth and little fingers?

Is it possible for you to imagine the volume of all of your fingers simultaneously and at the same time imagine the space between all of your fingers?

Can you imagine the volume of your shoulders, arms, hands, and fingers and at the same time imagine the space between your fingers and the distance or space between your arms?

Can you imagine that as you inhale naturally your breath fills your entire head, neck, shoulders, arms, hands, and fingers, and that as you exhale and as your breath leaves your body it leaves this entire region filled with space?

At the same time you're aware of the space inside this entire region, is it possible for you also to imagine the space around these regions; the space between your fingers; the space between your arms; the space around your arms, shoulders, neck, and head?

Can you imagine that as you continue to practice your experience will become more vivid and more effortless?

Can you imagine practicing this exercise at least twice daily?

4

The Domain of Pain Is Mainly in the Brain

That which is escaped now is pain to come.

—PROVERB

TRISH WAS A neurology nurse who switched careers and became a primary school teacher, a job she loved. In her third year of teaching kindergarten, though, she developed severe lower back pain—searing pain that radiated down her buttocks and legs and that sometimes kept her from work or, when she was at work, kept her from being with her students on the floor where they read and played. "I couldn't bend down and be spontaneous with the kids the way I wanted and in a way that I thought was important," she told me when she came for her initial evaluation. "There were many negatives on the job from that kind of pain."

Many of the people we see at our clinic have tried numerous other approaches to alleviate their pain, and they wind up coming to us because they are at the end of their rope. Trish was no exception. Pain medication, physical therapy, bed rest, special chairs, and cold compresses were among the things she had tried. These approaches gave her either limited relief or none at all. She seriously considered surgery but put it off, concerned about the risks involved.

Finally, when she was at her wit's end, a friend suggested brain-wave biofeedback and she came to see us. She filled out our standard eighty-question symptom checklist, and she was surprised to find she had not just one symptom (lower back pain) but fifteen different symptoms, some of which she hadn't thought much about. They included some sleeplessness and mild anxiety. In the Open-Focus model, many seemingly disparate symptoms, both physical and emotional problems, spring from the common source of RAS.

We like to have clients compare how they feel before and after Open-Focus training because often when the pain is lessened or gone completely, people forget the pain they were in, even if it was severe. We also ask clients to rank the frequency and severity of their bouts of pain before treatment, as a reference point.

Trish started practicing Open-Focus exercises with the neurofeedback equipment in our clinic, a system that teaches clients quickly to move out of narrow-focus attention, which constricts awareness, to a much more broadened awareness. We also had her work with the recorded exercises at home twice a day or more if possible.

"My symptoms started going away immediately with a couple of practice sessions," she told us later. "I was having pain that I ranked at 8, 9, or 10, with 10 meaning 'I cannot stand it anymore,' three or four hours a day every day. A month later, my pain was 1 or 2 or 3 once or twice a week. I could start assisting the kids again." After three months, Trish stopped having any back pain. If she noticed that her back was tense or painful, she could immediately move into Open Focus and head off the pain as it started to form, or sit down and listen to a recorded Open-Focus exercise. "The nurse part of me reacted to this with a lot of astonishment," she said. "I had come to rely on aspirin and other drugs to hold the pain off, but there are other ways to control pain."

Trish noticed other changes as she regularly started to broaden her awareness, things having nothing to do with pain. "My sensitivity to others improved," she said. "Before Open Focus, I had a way of pulling away from people, of going inside myself much of the time. Now I am not as remote from people." She also slept better, and her feelings of anxiety simply stopped.

Inspired by these results, she started to use some of the Open-Focus exercises in her classroom with her kids, and she noticed that as their awareness grew, they calmed somewhat and "became more sensitive to others in the class."

Trish was pleased she hadn't opted for surgery, as it turned out. Her back pain was not due to something wrong with a disk or a nerve, but was a problem that could, in the end, be traced back to how she paid attention.

Recognizing the Mind-Body Connection

Chronic pain is an epidemic in the United States, and one of the largest categories of pain is lower back pain. This in spite of the fact that only a small percentage of Americans do physically demanding labor. Yet back pain accounts for some 40 percent of compensation payments to disabled workers, and only the common cold causes more lost work time. Moreover, many people have no physical reason for back pain. In fact, one of the largest parts of our patient population are people whose pain does not respond to medical treatment.

Dr. John Sarno, who has written several books about the relationship between the mind and back pain, estimates that a very small percentage of people with back complaints have something physiologically wrong that causes the pain. For the majority, the source of pain lies in the complex relationship between the mind and the body. In Sarno's view, unexpressed negative emotions play a particularly important role in pain. We'll explore Sarno's theory in more detail later in this chapter, as we trace the emerging scientific understanding of the brain's role in pain. As I mentioned in the previous chapter, modern pain researchers are actively investigating the role of the mind, perceptions, and emotions in the pain experience.

The Gate-Control Theory of Pain

Modern research on a perception-based model of pain began with Ronald Melzack and Patrick Wall's gate-control theory. First published in the journal *Science* in 1965, this theory posits that the intensity of the pain we experience is the result not of the severity of our injury but of the interactions between pain-conducting and pain-inhibiting neurons along the neural pathway from the injury to the brain. Melzack and Wall proposed that pain-conducting neurons, or "transmitting cells," essentially open a "gate" for the pain signal to travel to the brain. However, they asserted there are also pain-inhibiting neurons that can close the pain gate, dialing down or stopping the pain signal.

The gate-control theory offered an explanation for why such things as rubbing a sore arm or a mother's kissing a child's scraped knee can make it feel better. These stimuli send a signal to the spine to close the gate to pain signals.

The most radical aspect of Melzack and Wall's theory—radical for the time anyway—was the claim that one of the major factors affecting the activation of pain-transmitting cells versus pain-inhibiting cells is our emotions. And they said that a physical injury need not ring the bell of pain at all—the mind alone could stop or mitigate the feeling of pain.

It was a seminal moment in the history of pain, and a radical departure from specificity. At the time, Dr. John Bonica, head of the University of Washington's Center for Pain Relief in Seattle, declared Melzack and Wall's theory "one of the major revolutions in our concept of pain over the last 100 years."

The gate-control theory accounted for the kinds of differences in pain perception that Henry Beecher had observed in the wounded soldiers and the civilians he interviewed. It also spurred interest in a host of new ways of investigating pain, investigations that included such issues as religious beliefs, moods, and the role of depression and anxiety in pain.

The Emerging Role of the Brain

In 1994, another milestone in the thinking about pain and emotions occurred. Dr. Frederick Lenz, a neurosurgeon at Johns Hopkins Hospital, was operating on the brain of a fully awake patient. The man had uncontrollable hand tremors that made his life extremely difficult. Even typing on a keyboard was a challenge. He sought help from Lenz, who treated such patients by destroying a few damaged cells in the brain's thalamus, cells that contribute to such tremors.

The patient also had a different, unassociated problem—severe panic disorders that caused chest pain, shortness of breath, and a pounding heart. A psychologist who had assessed the patient, though, thought the patient would do fine in surgery and the panic disorder would not cause complications.

With the patient fully conscious, under only a local anesthetic, Lenz drilled a hole in his skull. As he probed with a tiny electrical stimulator for the correct brain cells, he accidentally stimulated nearby cells that governed the patient's arm. Such stimulation in other patients caused a slight tingling in their arm. In this patient, however, it engendered a full-blown panic attack, causing feelings of suffocation and anxiety. Lenz was surprised. As the feelings died down, he disbelieved what had happened and tried stimulating the site again. Again, the discomfort of a panic attack rose up in the patient. Lenz moved on and cauterized the cells that caused the tremor.

Lenz was incredulous and remembered a similar occurrence. A woman with a history of heart pain, who came in for cauterization, also had a panic attack at the touch of the stimulator. These symptoms, which were wildly out of proportion to the stimulus and caused just a tingling sensation in most people, led Lenz to conclude that areas of the brain could become unstable in some people. "Lenz saw that areas of the brain governing ordinary sensations could become abnormally sensitized," wrote Dr. Atul Gawande, a neurosurgeon, in a 1998 article on this topic in the *New Yorker*.

Gawande went on to explain the significance of Lenz's discoveries as follows: "Lenz's finding suggests all pain is in the head. It is the brain that generates the pain experience, and it can do so even in the absence of external stimuli." This new understanding of the power of the brain in the pain experience finally explains the phenomenon of phantom limb pain. Areas of the brain associated with the missing limb can still, mistakenly, generate pain, probably because they are sensitized.

Lenz theorized the brain contains "neuromodules," circuits that fire throughout the brain that are similar to programs on a computer. Using these "programs" is how the brain binds together perceptual montages that include mood, senses, memory, and so forth from disparate regions of the brain. These highly sensitive neuromodules that govern, say, the lower back, in other words, are not fired to cause pain only when the back is physically injured. These networks of neurons can become so unstable they go haywire, and they can be set off by a host of triggers—moods, memories, stress, emotions, even seemingly nothing—and, in the complete absence of physical trauma, cause pain, even serious pain. The most significant factor at the root of pain, in other words, is a *hypersensitive, unstable brain*. This is the understanding of pain that lies at the heart of our Open-Focus approach. Open-Focus training engenders a more stable brain.

Tension Myositis Syndrome

A similar understanding of pain is found in the work of Dr. John Sarno, of the Rusk Institute of Rehabilitation Medicine at the New York University School of Medicine. Dr. Sarno posits that the cause of most back and joint pain is something he calls tension myositis syndrome, or TMS, a theory he has explained in his best-selling books *Healing Back Pain* and *Mind over Back Pain*.

Dr. Sarno maintains that we have a built-in defense mechanism against what is emotionally unpleasant and socially unacceptable—for example, shame, guilt, anger, anxiety, fear, and resentment. "The unconscious has been described as a kind of 'maximum security prison' where the brain keeps undesirable or dangerous feelings repressed," Dr. Sarno explains.

Since physical pain is more socially acceptable, the mind transfers the psychic pain to the body in order to give it an outlet. Where it shows up depends on different factors. If you are told typing can cause wrist pain, and you are a typist, that may be where the pain will arise. Not because the wrists are injured but because that's where the brain and mind decide pain should be manifested in a socially acceptable way. The brain/mind then reduces blood flow to the area. The reduction in blood flow to muscles, nerves, or tendons impedes normal function and eventually causes pain.

According to Dr. Sarno, becoming aware of the highly charged, negative emotions that lie at the root of pain is the most effective way to treat not only back pain but neck pain, knee pain, foot pain, hip pain, virtually any kind of pain, including the discomfort of irritable bowel syndrome, migraines, common allergies, and skin conditions such as eczema and psoriasis. Even fibromyalgia, he says, is a severe form of TMS.

Some people, of course, have been diagnosed with an abnormal disk or a torn rotator cuff as the cause of their pain. Dr. Sarno says that doctors can find structural abnormalities many places in the body to back up their diagnosis, even if those abnormalities are not causing the pain. He cites a study published in the *New England Journal of Medicine* in 1994 in which doctors did MRIs on ninety-eight people with no history of back pain and found that only about a third had normal disks. The other two-thirds had bulges and herniations, yet no pain. In other words, if you look for something that could be causing pain, you'll find it.

Though Dr. Sarno's theory differs in key ways from the Open-Focus model, I agree with his fundamental premise that highly charged emotions can play a major role in creating the experience of pain. In the Open-Focus model, however, it is not the feelings themselves that are the problem, but our resistance to those highly charged feelings that destabilizes the brain and causes the pain system to go haywire. Moreover, the content of those emotions does not matter as much as the way we attend to them. If difficult feelings are avoided through the strategy of narrow-focusing our attention away from the pain, this may buy us time but stresses the body and destabilizes the brain, sensitizing it to pain.

A growing body of research since the early 1990s in the field of psychosomatic medicine has shown that emotions can have profound physiological effects as well as psychological ones. Shame, for example, according to researchers, is a master emotion, a single type of emotional stress that causes many other kinds of inappropriate emotional responses, from anger to anxiety and even personality disorders such as narcissism. (Shame is different from guilt, which is about a particular act; shame is about the unworthiness of the whole self and so is more powerful.) Some researchers say it is the most difficult of emotions to discharge. And it is likely one of the main problems at the center of much of our experience of both physical and emotional pain, because it is the most powerful emotion, and resisting it causes the brain to become unstable. It's like trying to keep both the brake and the gas pedal depressed on a rapidly moving vehicle. We are repressing our painful emotions at the same time we are using our brain in everyday waking consciousness.

The Role of Memory

Another factor in how we now understand pain is a change in the psychological model of perception—how we deploy our senses in order to experience life. Dr. Richard Gregory, a professor emeritus of experimental psychology at the University of Bristol in the United Kingdom and the author of several books on perception, believes our internal world is far more important to our experiences than the external world. The reason we experience pain when there is no physical cause, or itching when there is nothing apparently causing the itch, is because most of what we experience in the world is based on past experience.

"Some 80% of fibres to the lateral geniculate nucleus relay station come downwards from the cortex, and only about 20% from the retinas," he writes in the *British Medical Journal*. "Sensations of consciousness are created by the brain. Perceptions are predictive hypotheses, based on knowledge stored from the past." In other words, most of our perception, including the perception of pain, is generated *internally*.

Rigid Attention Syndrome (RAS)

I know that it's difficult for people who have a chronically aching shoulder or back to accept the fact that the pain is not in the aching tissue but in their mind and brain. Many of my patients say, "It hurts so much, it has to be in the muscle." Or, "Why would I create the pain?" Or they may feel they are somehow being blamed for the chronic pain, even though they have no idea what is going on. They might think that it's akin to someone saying the pain is all in their head. But it's not. The pain is real and physical—the neurons in the brain, after all, are under tremendous pressure from stress chemicals. And it's not all in the brain. The muscles are very tense, and nerves are impacted—they are just tensed for emotional reasons, not purely physical ones.

In an emotional situation, I believe, as we start to feel the discomfort of fear traveling throughout the body, we unconsciously and reflexively tense muscles to keep from feeling the fear. These muscles then stay somewhat tense. We labor to keep the pain distant from consciousness by narrow-focus aversion from feeling. We objectify the pain in both brain and body. This causes it to hurt more, which further activates the sympathetic autonomic nervous system, our fight-or-flight system, which causes arousal, which, in turn, causes more pain. Back pain can activate the entire nervous system in this kind of loop, and it can go on for years.

Tensing muscles or nerves or tendons as part of the act of repressing high-energy emotional feelings causes a reduction in blood flow and oxygen to certain susceptible areas, which, in turn, causes muscle contractions and nerve pain.

This rigid attention theory explains the epidemic of chronic pain in our culture and the fact that much, if not most, of this pain has no detectable physical origin. It's a behavioral loop, and we can use Trish's back pain as an example. She learned to narrow-focus in childhood to avoid feelings of fear—which she held back with her muscles, in her stomach, and in other parts of her body. Her anxiety accumulated from a combination of events, but nothing momentous. Almost everyone does this, and resisting these feelings is often so successful we don't know we are doing it.

These feelings, if left unacknowledged and unaddressed, can eventually surface as pain of some kind. Then the pain, in turn, causes us to narrow-focus on distractions, from television to the Internet or a range of things. By using narrow-focus avoidance to hold back our unwanted thoughts and feelings, our nervous system goes into overarousal, creating muscle tension and blood flow disturbances, which lead to the production of auxiliary pain. In Trish's case, it was back pain.

Modern medicine does not, by and large, acknowledge that the mind can so profoundly influence the body, and so doctors often ignore the connection between pain and emotions. Few in the medical profession take this model of pain seriously. Even many therapists, who are confronted with the mind-body connection daily, don't understand that we feel emotional stress with our body and not just in our mind.

While chronic pain has a physical component and treating the muscle by stretching or with medical intervention helps, it is the smaller part of the pain puzzle. Treating only the body can leave behind a neural platform upon which the pain can rebuild itself. That's what we see with phantom limb pain.

Dr. Sarno has no treatment regimen for his approach, other than for people to read his books and understand where their pain comes from—knowledge is the penicillin, he says. Some talk therapists also approach physical pain this way and have pain patients discuss their fear and anxiety and anger in a therapeutic setting.

I have no doubt that psychotherapy can help people recognize emotional issues, reduce the "charge" of these emotions, and alleviate physical pain and distress. My wife and colleague, Susan Shor Fehmi, has been a talk therapist and a biofeedback therapist for more than thirty years and has seen much release of physical pain with the talking cure. There's a more direct way, though, which she now uses. She helps her clients to dissolve their pain with Open Focus before discussing the pain's psychological origins.

Remember, the Open-Focus model suggests that it's not the type of emotion but the way we attend to it that matters. It's an intensity problem, of sorts, and we need to reduce the charge of those emotions. We do that by shifting how we pay attention both to the world in and around us and specifically to the emotions themselves.

Exercise

General Training in Open Focus

The purpose of this exercise is to develop a deep sense of space in, around, and through the body to facilitate the release of tension and pain.

An audio recording of this exercise can be found on the enclosed CD, track 2. For information on how to download an audio recording of this exercise, please see page 183.

If you are reading this exercise aloud, remember to allow fifteen seconds between the end of one question and the beginning of the next question. We recommend initially practicing this exercise with eyes closed.

Guiding Questions

Can you imagine that no effort is required to listen to or imagine what follows?

Can you imagine what it would be like not to concentrate—neither focusing upon nor focusing away from listening to the following questions?

Can you imagine that your imagination is very subtle and effortless and includes all your senses, not just visualization?

Can you imagine letting your multisensory imagination respond however it may as you listen to the following questions?

Can you imagine letting your awareness center itself on body feeling without excluding the senses of hearing, seeing, tasting, smelling, mental activity, and the sense of time?

Is it possible for you to imagine what it would feel like to sense the three-dimensional presence of your thumbs?

Is it possible for you now to imagine what it would feel like to experience the presence of your thumbs even more sensitively than you already are?

Is it possible for you now to imagine what it would feel like if you were already experiencing your index fingers (the fingers closest to your thumbs) as intimately as you are sensing your thumbs?

Can you imagine experiencing the three-dimensional presence of your thumbs and index fingers simultaneously?

Is it possible for you to imagine what it would feel like if you could experience the presence of your thumb and index finger on both hands and also sense the absence between your thumb and index finger on each hand simultaneously?

Can you imagine that the sense of absence in the space between your thumb and index finger can be experienced as intimately and as sensitively as you experience the sense of presence of your thumbs and index fingers?

Can you imagine the fact that your fingers are made up of atoms of matter? An atom of matter is composed of a nucleus with electrons revolving about it. The nucleus of an atom is two hundred thousand times smaller than the diameter of the atom. The electrons are many times smaller than the nucleus. In other words, can you imagine the reality that an atom of matter consists of millions of times more space than solid matter?

Can you imagine that your fingers are made up of atoms, clouds of tiny particles revolving around one another, floating in a vast space, a space that flows from outside your fingers through the spaces between the particles, in every direction?

Can you imagine that your thumbs and index fingers are clouds of particles floating in space, right where they actually are, surrounded by space and permeated by space?

Can you imagine feeling the space even more subtly and intimately?

Can you imagine experiencing your middle fingers as intimately as your thumbs and index fingers—filled with space, surrounded by space, permeated by space?

Can you imagine experiencing your ring fingers filled with space—clouds of particles, permeated by space?

Can you imagine experiencing your little fingers as fogs of feeling, permeated by space?

Can you imagine experiencing the space surrounding and permeating the clouds of feeling of all your fingers simultaneously?

Can you imagine letting this sensation of absence and presence serve as a model for experiencing other portions of your body?

For example, is it possible for you to imagine that your hands are filled with space, surrounded by space, permeated by space, and can you imagine experiencing the space of your hands and fingers as intimately as you experience the space of your fingers alone?

Can you imagine what it would feel like to experience your feet and toes as clouds of particles floating in space—as intimately as you now experience the space permeating your hands and fingers?

Can you imagine experiencing your wrists and forearms, your elbows and upper arms, filled with space, surrounded by space, just as sensitively as you experience the space of your hands and fingers?

Can you imagine experiencing your arms, hands and fingers, and your feet and toes, and now your ankles, lower legs, knees, and upper legs as clouds of feeling, permeated by space, as intimately and subtly as you feel the space of your hands and fingers and feet and toes?

Can you imagine experiencing the three-dimensional

presence of your shoulders and the region between your shoulders as being filled with space, surrounded by space, permeated by space? Can you imagine experiencing this as intimately and as subtly as you feel the space of your hands and fingers, feet and toes, arms and legs?

Can you imagine experiencing your hips, the region between your hips, and your buttocks as a fog of feeling permeated by space?

Can you imagine experiencing your abdomen and navel and the region between these and your back, and your internal organs (including reproductive, eliminative, and digestive organs) as mists of feeling permeated by space?

Can you imagine what it would feel like to sense your chest and back, the region between your ribs, and all the organs inside your rib cage (including your lungs, heart, and esophagus) permeated by space—clouds of particles floating in space?

Is it possible for you to imagine what it would feel like to experience your neck and your throat filled with space, surrounded by space, permeated by space?

Is it possible for you to imagine experiencing your whole body from the neck down as a cloud of particles surrounded by space, permeated by space—just as sensitively as you experience the space of your hands and fingers, feet and toes?

Can you imagine that as you inhale and exhale naturally, you can feel the space inside your entire respiratory system?

Can you imagine that as you inhale naturally, you can experience your breath flowing up behind and around your eyes?

Is it possible for you to imagine that your lips are clouds of feeling filled with space, permeated by space, kissing space?

Is it possible for you to imagine what it would feel like to experience your tongue, teeth and gums, jaw and chin, cheeks and cheekbones, and the regions between them filled with space, permeated by space—just as sensitively and as intimately as you experience the space of your lips, hands and fingers, feet and toes?

Can you imagine the space inside your ears and the space between your ears, as intimately as you experience the space inside and between your lips, hands and fingers, feet and toes?

Can you imagine the space between your eyes and the space between each eye and the nearest temple?

Can you imagine what it would feel like to sense the space touching and permeating your eyes and eyelids, in front, behind, on the sides, and the space above and below your eyes, as intimately as you experience the space touching and permeating your lips and fingers?

Can you imagine experiencing your eyebrows, forehead, temples, the sides of your head, the back of your head, and the tip of your head as being touched and permeated by space?

Can you imagine experiencing the space between your eyelids and the back of your head?

Can you imagine now sensing your whole body simultaneously as a cloud of particles, a fog of feeling, including a mist of emotion, floating in space, permeated by space—just as sensitively as you experience the space of your hands, fingers, feet, and toes?

Can you imagine feeling also the space in the whole room—in addition to the space permeating you, other people, and the objects in the room?

In addition to feeling the space, can you imagine visualizing the space in the whole room?

Can you imagine hearing the three-dimensional silence in the space of the room, the silence out of which sounds arise, the silence in which sounds exist and into which they fade?

Can you imagine space surrounding and permeating the thoughts, visual images, and internal dialogues of your mind as space permeates and surrounds your entire body, feelings, and emotions?

Can you imagine seeing space, feeling space, hearing silence, and experiencing the space in your mind, all simultaneously?

Can you imagine experiencing also the sensory space in which tastes and smells occur?

Is it possible for you now to experience the space of these six senses simultaneously and equally? Can you imagine feeling space, seeing space, hearing silence, experiencing mind-space, and the space in which tastes and smells occur?

Can you imagine now including within your awareness a seventh space: the space in which you simultaneously sense past, present, and future time—a space called time-lessness?

Can you imagine that the aspect of awareness that is simultaneously and effortlessly witnessing these seven spaces is also a cloud surrounded and permeated by space?

Can you imagine that this cloud of awareness can now diffuse throughout your experience of these seven spaces, witnessing these spaces from inside these spaces, immersing awareness throughout these spaces, experiencing these spaces more intimately, more subtly, more sensitively, equally, and simultaneously?

Is it possible for you to imagine participating in your everyday activities with the awareness you are experiencing now—that is, in Open Focus?

Can you imagine practicing these exercises at least twice daily?

5

The Role of Attention in Pain

The mind is its own place, and in itself
Can make a heav'n of hell, a hell of heav'n.

—Milton

From the beginning of our lives, pain is nature's alarm system, drawing our awareness to a place in the body where something is amiss so that we can attend to it and solve whatever the problem may be. Some researchers have found that we can alleviate pain powerfully by drawing awareness away from the source of pain to something outside of the body. In this chapter, we'll explore the redirection of attention in the treatment of pain—and how this contrasts with the Open-Focus approach.

Attention Diversion in Pain Treatment

SnowWorld is the name of an imaginary place that is part of a therapeutic virtual-reality (VR) system used by patients at the University of Washington Harborview Burn Center in Seattle during wound care. The power of attention in pain relief is being researched here.

For people who have been severely burned, peeling off old bandages that cover their wounds is always extremely painful. Even morphine only dulls the excruciating pain. Wearing goggles that create total immersion in a cold, snowy world, however, enables patients to enter a space nearly free of pain.

In one study, researchers placed two subjects undergoing wound care in a virtual-reality environment. Each subject watched a standard video game on a television during the process of bandage removal. In the second part of the study, they wore goggles that allowed them to travel through the cool and immersive all-encompassing virtual world and participate in a game in which they had to shoot snowballs at attackers.

In this study, published in the journal *Pain* in 2000, one patient thought of his pain 95 percent of the time while playing the video game, but just 2 percent of the time while his attention was far more fully diverted and engaged by his actions in virtual-reality gear. The other patient went from thinking of his pain 91 percent of the time while watching the video to 36 percent in virtual reality.

"Pain perception has a strong psychological component," writes Dr. Hunter Hoffman, the creator of the system. "The same incoming pain signal can be interpreted as painful or not, depending on what the patient is thinking. Pain requires conscious attention. Being drawn into another world drains a lot of attentional resources, leaving less attention available to process pain signals." He continues, "Conscious attention is like a spotlight. Usually it is focused on the pain and wound care. We are luring that spotlight into the virtual world. Rather than having pain as the focus of their attention, for many patients in VR, the wound care becomes more of an annoyance, distracting them from their primary goal of exploring the virtual world."

Virtual-world therapy is not the only place where attention diversion is being used to manage pain—it's widely used in a number of other ways. In Lamaze childbirth, for example, women are given breathing and other exercises to keep them from focusing their attention on the pain.

Our culture in fact unwittingly diverts our attention from our pain much of the time. Consider our emotional pain, such as anxiety or depression. As feelings of anxiety rise, we unconsciously look for effective distractions. We might choose something that rivets our attention away from the anxiety, such as a fast-paced movie or thrilling video game. These can help us to escape emotional chaos, anxiousness, or any kind of unpleasantness from within (or without, such as a painful family life). The more strongly something holds our interest, the more effectively it functions as an anxiety-management tool. Many people have focused their attention away from unwanted feelings for so long, they may not even know they are still trying to resist them.

Diversionary strategies are often overused to the point of addiction—compulsive use of television, sex, gambling, travel, shopping, video games, loud music, alcohol, and working long hours are often distraction strategies to keep our attention on something besides our emotional discomfort or pain. At some point, however, pain often becomes so great that diversionary tactics don't work. (Think back to my unsuccessful effort to distract my attention away from the intense kidney-stone pain by bending my thumb or pinching myself.) If attention aversion works, we'll keep using it until it stops being effective or becomes too expensive. When one type of diversion stops working, we'll find a more potent distraction, if we can.

Diversion is essentially what the virtual-reality therapists are doing with physical pain. There is a finite pool of attention, they say, and the more successfully that pool is diverted to a virtual world, the less attention is available for feeling the pain of wound care. However, there's another way to use attention that is beyond diversion, one that lasts beyond the time when our attention is diverted.

The Role of Attention in Pain

Alternatives to Attention Diversion

Whether we realize it or not, we pay attention to physical pain (as well as emotional pain) in narrow-objective focus, fighting our pain and trying to keep it at a distance. Remember that narrow focus is the emergency mode of attending, and it raises arousal. Meanwhile, objective focus separates us from the object of attention. Sometimes we pay attention that way consciously, but most often we are holding the pain in narrow-objective attention unconsciously. Even as you read this and even if you have no awareness that you are doing this with your pain, you are. The problem with narrow focus as an avoidance strategy is that it raises arousal levels in the nervous system, tenses muscles, and can make the pain worse.

Evolution, however, did not give us pain without giving us anti-pain: we are equipped with an innate and robust normalizing mechanism in the human body, accessed and operated not by diverting our attention but by broadening our scope of awareness and becoming more subtle and sensitive in how we pay attention.

We can go from a removed, objective attentional posture to an immersed one. We can go from a narrow beam of attention to a broader, more diffuse beam, something like a camera that we can focus on just one person or open the lens and take in a whole crowd of people. It seems subtle, but learning to move from a narrow-objective focus to a diffuse-immersed one has a huge impact. And it is not just a temporary fix—it's one that we can learn to use repeatedly and make last.

Broadening and immersing our attention this way encourages the brain to produce more of the slower, more rhythmic brainwave frequencies associated with healing, balance, and well-being. These changes cause all of our psychological and physiological systems to respond, calming the sympathetic nervous system's over-arousal and engaging the parasympathetic nervous system. We become immersed and open once again, like the house cat that has finished chasing its prey and is now recovering from the attack.

Blood flow returns to normal as our muscles relax, as well as the gastrointestinal system and the skin and other areas. Respiratory and heart rates decrease. Adrenaline and cortisol levels return to normal. In short, moving out of narrow-objective attention increases the brain's production of alpha brain waves and engenders a powerful normalization response.

It's a great wonder—one I believe that has largely escaped scientific notice—that a simple shift in how we pay attention results in profound changes in brain activity that reflect nervous system function.

It hasn't, however, completely escaped scientific notice. Several studies, in such journals as the *Archives of Psychiatry, Headache Quarterly,* and the *International Journal of Clinical and Experimental Hypnosis,* have found that just increasing the production of alpha brain waves—which comes with a shift in attention—causes a reduction in the patient reports of many kinds of chronic pain, including migraines, tension headaches, and back pain. Alpha training has also been shown to greatly reduce anxiety and depression and to reduce symptoms associated with post-traumatic stress disorder. In a 1984 study published in *Psychosomatic Medicine,* alpha training was associated with "clear thinking."

In one of my own studies, conducted with a colleague and published in the *Journal of Neurotherapy* in 2001, we found that alpha worked to reduce stress-induced pain. We analyzed 132 patients who engaged in Open-Focus and synchrony training, and found that more than 90 percent reported alleviation of stress-induced pain, from joint pain to headaches to gastrointestinal problems.

Changes in attention might also be behind the placebo effect, the well-documented ability of sugar pills given as part of a drug study, for example, to heal serious illness. When patients are unknowingly given a sugar pill during a drug study, they naturally shift from worry over their illness to hopeful expectation that it will be cured. They let go of a narrow-objective attention to their symptoms and open their awareness as they begin to look for signs of improvement. They unconsciously release their lock on narrow-objective focus and take on a more diffuse-immersed form of attention, which increases alpha brain-wave activity, which in turn promotes healing.

Diffuse attention also creates a larger field of awareness in which our pain takes up a smaller percentage of the space. We become aware of more than just our pain or discomfort, and sometimes the pain simply disappears into this much larger ocean of awareness.

The question then becomes, how do we consciously expand our awareness so that it can dwarf and diffuse the pain? The answer is: nothing, and by that I mean no-thing, nothingness. Let me explain.

6

The Miracle of Space

Nothing is more real than nothing.

—Samuel Beckett

In chapter 1, I mentioned my early experiments at the Brain Research Institute at UCLA. In the 1960s, as an assistant professor at the State University of New York at Stony Brook, I was searching for a way to help people enter an alpha state (the EEG signature of diffuse-immersed attention) for the relief of stress. I experimented often on myself trying to produce more alpha activity.

After twelve sessions of almost two hours each, engaging in futile attempts to get my alpha to increase, I gave up and accepted the fact that it was simply impossible for me to create alpha on demand. Ironically, the second I gave up and accepted my failure, the EEG registered a significant increase in alpha amplitudes and duration. I realized I had been trying too hard. By surrendering, I slipped into the effortless, interested attention that had eluded me all along.

Earlier in the book, I mentioned how my muscles softened, arthritis pain, tensions, and mild anxiety dissolved. This makes sense from an evolutionary point of view. Chronic anxiety and pain are not the natural state of human beings or necessarily the result of a brain that is somehow fundamentally flawed—they are the result of "operator error." When people learn to operate their central nervous system the way I believe it was designed to be used, through voluntary changes in attention, mind and body systems don't break down as often and become more stable and resilient. We know we can—and must—maintain our own health with nutrition, exercise, and diet, but we must, most critically, maintain it through the way we pay attention.

Remember that after my training, I perceived larger scenes without overfocusing on any one element and with much less effort? It wasn't just visual. It's hard to describe, but my awareness of the room I was in, my sense of it, was also much bigger and much more vivid. Sometimes I filled the room up with my awareness. It was my first glimpse of Open-Focus attention.

My production of alpha during the session caused a multisensory attention shift from a narrow-objective attention to a wide, diffuse one and moved me from an attention state in which I felt separated from experience to a more sensitive absorption with the world around me. Second, the EEG showed that when we attend in full Open Focus, not only do we produce alpha but we produce a very specific kind, called phase-synchronous alpha.

Synchrony means that a very large number of cells are working rhythmically together—an especially powerful type of synergistic neural activity. The effect of synchrony is greater than the sum of its parts. A laser beam is powerful enough to use as a cutting torch, yet it is only light. But it is powerful because the light waves are in phase, meaning their waveforms are increasing and decreasing in unison. Dr. William Tiller, a professor emeritus of engineering at Stanford, writes, "If we could somehow take the same number of photons emitted by [a 60-watt] lightbulb per second and orchestrate their emission to be in phase with each other . . . the energy density at the surface of the lightbulb would be thousands to millions of times higher than the present photon energy density at the surface of the sun."

A number of published studies of veteran meditators have demonstrated that alpha synchrony can greatly diminish or eliminate many different kinds of pain. In 2009, researchers published a study in the journal *Psychosomatic Medicine* involving thirteen meditators and thirteen individuals who didn't practice meditation. They pressed a heating plate to the legs of both groups and found that the meditators, even when they were not meditating, could tolerate heat up to the maximum of 53 degrees Celsius (127 degrees Fahrenheit), while the nonmeditators could only tolerate temperatures well below that.

In another 2009 study in the journal *Pain,* scientist at the University of North Carolina at Charlotte found that just twenty minutes of meditation for three days can reduce a subject's perception of the intensity of pain, even in subjects who have never meditated before.

Other studies, including one published in the journal *Science* in 1978, have shown alpha enhancement to be effective for different kinds of emotional pain, from anxiety to depression.

After I realized the tremendous potential of in-phase alpha, the focus of my research shifted to finding a way to help produce those brain waves as quickly as possible and on demand. It had taken me twenty-four hours over twelve days to learn how to let go and increase alpha amplitude and duration. That was too long for it to be effective as a therapy. Many people would end participation before they experienced relief from stress and pain. Besides, there was no way to verbally instruct someone in how to do it. It took experience, trial and error.

In 1971, I exposed student volunteers to a number of stimuli as their EEG was monitored to see which ones produced the most phase-synchronous alpha. Some were asked to visualize peaceful pastoral scenes and other relaxing imagery. One day I introduced a twenty-item relaxation inventory to undergraduate students.

During the first few questions—imagine a waterfall or a dew-drop on a rose petal, for example—their EEG manifested little change. Then, in the middle of the inventory, the students were asked, "Can you imagine the space between your eyes?" Boom. Their brains produced abundant phase-synchronous alpha. The second question was, "Can you imagine the space between your ears?" Again, instantly abundant high-amplitude alpha appeared. No other question or imagery brought about such profound changes in the EEG as the experience and awareness of space, nothingness, or absence.

During further research, I found that using this "objectless imagery" almost always elicits large amplitude and prolonged periods of phase-synchronous alpha activity very quickly. In other words, experiencing space is a shortcut to alpha-wave activity. Nothing is far more than nothing. "No-thing" is a robust healer of the human central nervous system and critical to our health and well-being. Space is unique among perceptions because space, silence, and timelessness cannot be grasped fully by our attention as a separate object.

The awareness of space slips through and permeates your senses. Seeing, hearing, tasting, feeling, smelling, and thinking of space, bathing in it on every level, while experiencing a sense of timelessness, is a powerful way to relax the nervous system, the most powerful and most rapid way I know.

For example, can you imagine feeling the space in the whole room you are in right now?

Did you let go or open your attention in response to the question?

Exploring the Surprising Power of Space, Silence, and Timelessness

I discovered the robust effects of the awareness of space on the central nervous system on my own, with the help of brain synchrony, but I was certainly not the first to discover these effects. There are numerous examples of space and nothingness as a component of meditation. The Japanese have a philosophy of *ma*, cultivating the awareness of objects as well as the space between them. One Eastern mystic, Master Hakuin, wrote that it was important to "attain a state of mind in which even though surrounded by crowds of people, it is as if you were alone in a field extending for tens of thousands of miles." All of these different approaches probably yield slower cortical rhythms and dial down the central nervous system.

Work by several researchers, meanwhile, would later show that phase-synchronous alpha is the hallmark of veteran meditators. What I'd done, in effect, was discover the physiological outcome or essence of Eastern meditation practice, and described it in the language of Western psychology and science.

Since a sustained awareness of space is key to Open Focus, I recorded a series of exercises to guide people through different kinds of objectless space imagery, asking them to imagine space extending to the walls, ceiling, floor, and beyond in every direction, or asking them to imagine space in and around their eyes, neck and head, and hands. Or asking them to imagine space in, around, and through their pain. When people imagine space, and center their awareness on it, the brain responds immediately, dropping into whole-brain synchronous alpha.

It's more than just a general response. When we imagine space around specific parts of the body—the stomach, for example—it targets the release of pain and tension to the specific area, as well as providing a general release.

Add neurofeedback equipment—sensors placed on the scalp that detect when the brain is producing alpha—and people can change very quickly. In the 1960s, I designed a feedback system with five sensors on the scalp connected to a device that "rewards" people with light and sound feedback when they produce phase-synchronous alpha. With this feedback, people quickly learn to produce alpha activity, whereas some meditators might take years to accomplish this.

What is the physiological mechanism that explains why imagining space and silence has this sudden and powerful effect on the brain? Part of it may be that the brain is very busy when it is making sense out of the objects in the world. When it is processing sense objects—either physical or imagined—it uses desynchronized activity in order to make that processing possible. Electrical signals that bind together different regions of the brain move at speeds exceeding a hundred miles an hour.

When the mind is asked to imagine space, however, there is "no thing" to grasp, objectify, and make sense of, and the brain is allowed to quit its rapid processing and take a vacation. Cortical rhythms slow quickly into alpha, and a racing brain and mind become a stress-reducing brain and a quiet mind. Space seems to reset neural networks affected by stress, returning them to their original, fully balanced functioning.

When we are well trained in flexible attention, we can readily move into alpha activity when emergency functions aren't needed, just as the cat does after its hunt. The cat fixes on a single object of prey, or chases that object down and kills it, if need be, in narrow-objective focus. During the hunt, the mouse is foreground, and everything else is relegated to the periphery or background of attention. Narrow focus played its role—it induced a surge in adrenaline, increasing blood flow to the large muscle groups and increasing heart rate to support stalking, chasing, and the takedown.

When the chase ends, the cat's attention moves out of narrow focus toward a diffuse focus in which there is no longer a strong distinction between figure and ground, breaking with emergency function. The cat is now resting in every sense of the word, seeing everything equally and simultaneously. This diffuse-immersed attention represents not only a break with emergency function but a process the cat can engage to actually reverse the effects of stress from the hunt.

Exercise

Localizing Pain

This exercise is designed to help you discover where in your body the worst of your pain is located. By finding its exact location or center, you take a powerful step toward being able to merge with it and dissolve it, using the "Dissolving Pain" exercise, as well as the other exercises that follow it. If you already know where your pain is centered in the body, it is not necessary to do this exercise.

Remember to allow fifteen seconds between the end of one question and the beginning of the next question.

Guiding Questions

Can you imagine already being more fully in Open Focus than you ever have been?

Can you imagine experiencing all your senses simultaneously and equally, centering your attention upon feeling the presence of your body and mind, and the space they occupy, and the three-dimensional space around them, to infinity in every direction?

Can you imagine resting in all your feeling experience in this moment?

Can you imagine scanning your present experience for any current feeling, emotion, sensation, pain, or attitude? Examples include tension, impatience, annoyance, fatigue, boredom, confusion, restlessness, anger, fear, loneliness, guilt, depression, anxiety, or any other feeling that is present in this moment at any level of intensity.

Can you imagine choosing the most intense present feeling and centering your attention upon this feeling? If anxiety, for example, is the most intense experience, then the causes of this anxiety or your reactions to this anxiety are not the same feeling as the anxiety itself. For example, the reactions of bracing, tensing, sweating, a pounding heart, or hyperventilation, if present, are not the feeling of anxiety itself. Center your attention only upon the feeling of the most intense anxiety itself, and imagine feeling precisely where it is located in your body.

Is it possible for you to imagine feeling that portions or percentages of this experience are localized in specific regions of your body? Can you, for example, sense whether half or two-thirds or even all of your most intense experience is localized in one or more specific regions of your body? If, at any time during the course of this exercise, you feel that all of the most intense experience is felt in one or more specific parts of your body, then practice one of the "Dissolving Pain" exercises to diffuse the most intense of your localized experiences.

Can you imagine that the unlocalized portion of the most intense experience may be free-floating in space, or may be an all-over-body feeling in space, or may be sensed as a feeling in mind-space?

Can you imagine that if you cannot successfully localize your pain in your body, then it is considered unlocalized?

Can you imagine maintaining a feeling of space, surrounding and permeating mind and body, extending to the walls, ceiling, and floor of the room you are in, throughout the exercise?

Can you now imagine centering your attention on the unlocalized experience while letting the body-localized portion of this same experience remain present in the background of your attention?

Is it possible for you to imagine basking in the feeling of your unlocalized experience in a more absorbed way and more sensitively? As you do so, can you now sense where some or all of your pain experience is located within your body?

Can you imagine sensing what percentage of your most intense experience remains unlocalized at this moment?

Again, can you imagine merging with and bathing in the feeling of this remaining unlocalized experience even more subtly and completely, while sensing where this feeling is located in your body during this merging process?

Again, can you imagine feeling what percentage of your most intense experience continues to remain unlocalized?

Can you imagine more totally immersing yourself in and merging with any remaining unlocalized experience, while at the same time sensing where this unlocalized experience is centered in your body?

Again, can you imagine feeling the percentage of your most intense experience that still remains unlocalized?

Can you imagine rating on a 0–10 scale how intense the unlocalized experience is compared to the possible presence of the same feeling in your feet?

Can you imagine rating which is stronger, your unlocalized experience or the possible presence of the same feeling in your legs?

Can you imagine rating the strength of your unlocalized experience as compared to the present feeling in your hip joints and buttocks? Which is stronger?

Can you imagine rating the intensity of your unlocalized experience as compared to the present feeling in your lower GI system and lower back? Which is more intense?

Can you imagine rating the intensity of the unlocalized experience as compared to the present feeling in your lower abdomen and reproductive organs?

Can you imagine now rating the intensity of the unlocalized experience as compared to the feeling present in your stomach and waist region, including the feeling present in your middle back?

Can you imagine now rating the intensity of the unlocalized experience as compared to the same feeling present in your solar plexus and diaphragm?

Can you imagine rating the intensity of the unlocalized experience as compared to the feeling present in your rib cage, heart, chest, and upper back?

Can you now imagine rating the unlocalized experience as compared to the feeling present in your respiratory system, including the feeling present in your nose, sinuses, pharynx, larynx, trachea, bronchial tubes, and lungs?

Can you imagine rating the intensity of the unlocalized experience as compared to the feeling present in your hands and arms?

Can you now imagine comparing the intensity of the unlocalized experience to the feeling in your shoulders?

Can you imagine comparing the intensity of the unlocalized experience to the feeling in your face and eyes?

Can you imagine comparing the intensity of the unlocalized experience to the feeling present in your head?

Can you now imagine comparing the intensity of the feeling in your hands to the intensity of the feeling of presence of your feet?

Can you imagine comparing the intensity of the feeling in your arms to the feeling of your legs?

Can you imagine comparing the feeling in your hips to the feeling in your shoulders and sensing where these feelings are more intense than the unlocalized experience?

Can you imagine comparing the experience of your lower back to that of your middle back and sensing in which place the feeling is more intense than the unlocalized experience?

Can you imagine comparing the feeling in your buttocks to that in your reproductive organs and sensing where the feeling is more intense than the unlocalized experience?

Can you imagine comparing the feeling of intensity in your stomach to that in your solar plexus and sensing where the feeling is more intense than the unlocalized experience?

Can you imagine comparing the feeling in your chest to that in your upper back and sensing in which of these body parts the feeling is more intense than the unlocalized experience?

Can you imagine now comparing the feeling in your heart to the feeling in your throat and sensing where the feeling is more intense than the unlocalized experience?

Can you imagine now comparing the feeling in your neck to the feeling in your jaw and sensing where the feeling is more clearly similar to the unlocalized experience?

Can you imagine now comparing the feeling in your mouth to the feeling in your eyes and sensing where the feeling is more intense than the unlocalized experience?

Can you imagine now comparing your face to the sides of your head and sensing where the feeling is more intense than the unlocalized experience?

Can you imagine comparing the feeling present in the top of your head to the feeling present in the back of your head and sensing which of these two feelings is more intense than the unlocalized experience?

Once again, can you imagine feeling how much of the original pain experience is localized in your body? Is 100 percent of it now localized in your body, or does some of it remain unlocalized, that is, in your mind?

Can you now imagine centering your attention on the most intense body-localized portion of the chosen experience, sensing its shape and the space around it, and the space it occupies, while feeling the space in the whole room?

Can you imagine what it would feel like if this awareness, which is you, was already merged with the body experience, feeling this experience from inside the space that it occupies?

Can you imagine feeling the most intense experience, which is now localized in one or more parts of your body?

If less than 100 percent is localized, then can you imagine repeating this exercise once or twice in order to fully localize your chosen experience in your body?

If all or most of your chosen experience is localized, then can you imagine using the "Dissolving Pain" exercise to dissolve your localized experience?

7

The Full Range of Attention

*A man once asked Zen Master Ikkyu, "Please write some-
thing of great wisdom for me." The Zen master picked up
his brush and wrote one word: "Attention." The man was
not satisfied and asked for something more. Ikkyu then
wrote, "Attention. Attention. Attention."*

—TRADITIONAL ZEN TEACHING STORY

FOR TWO YEARS, Michael, an executive coach, suffered migraines. Every night the pain would arise, pressing on the sides of
his head, pain so intense it made sleep difficult and sometimes
impossible. His doctor prescribed medication, but it didn't help
much. At a conference of executive coaches in 2007, Martha Beck,
a columnist for *O* magazine, told him about my book *The Open-
Focus Brain*. He immediately ordered the book, and by the time
he arrived home from the conference, it was waiting for him with
the included CD of recorded exercises.

That evening the familiar pain started coming on. By the time
Michael got the exercise ready to play, he was in serious pain
from the migraine. "It was hard to focus, I was in so much pain,"

he said. But he managed to get through the general Open-Focus exercise and was surprised at how much it helped alleviate the pain. "Within about thirty minutes of practice, I started to feel the vise grip in my head and around my eyes start to dissipate," he told me. The next night he was ready, and as soon as the pain started forming on the sides of his head, he listened to the exercise. As he listened, he could feel the pain starting to subside, and then he fell asleep. "It was great, because for months it had been difficult to sleep." He slept through the night and woke up with no headache.

"I was skeptical that a book could actually help with physical conditions," he says, "but I have been surprised by how effective the Open-Focus exercises are. They diminish or eliminate pain for days at a time."

Michael says that at first he listened to the exercises only when he started to feel a migraine coming on, and this prevented the headache from forming. Then, when he began doing the General Training exercises every day, the migraines stopped completely and he was able to get a good night's sleep. When I last spoke with him, he hadn't had a migraine in six months.

He also had serious back pain, and the Open-Focus training helped that as well. "It doesn't make my back pain go away," he said. "But Open Focus helps me manage it."

All of this pain relief came from practicing exercises that simply moved Michael out of narrow-objective attention—indicating that much of this pain was the product of RAS, or rigid attention syndrome.

It seems incredible that an open style of attention can be so effective in alleviating pain of all kinds, physical and emotional. But the many hundreds of clients I have treated over the years have all benefited any number of ways just from basic attention training—moving out of narrow-objective focus. Sometimes, as in Michael's case, just thirty minutes of attention training can make a noticeable difference.

How can simply changing the way we attend resolve so many different kinds of pain? Remember that narrow-objective attention maintains the fight-or-flight response and tamps down some physiological systems that aren't needed for an emergency—immune and digestive functions, for example, get put on the back burner. Meanwhile, narrow-objective attention amps up other systems that are needed in an emergency, such as the speed of the strategic mind and the heart and respiratory rates.

As a response to stress, blood is routed away from the digestive system. This is why emotional stress can cause many digestive problems, everything from irritable bowel syndrome to constipation. The pallor associated with emergency ("You look as pale as a ghost") is due to blood being shunted away from the skin, which is why *overuse* of narrow-objective attention and prolonged stress can lead to itching, eczema, and other dermatological problems.

During an emergency, large muscles tense, preparing for an attack or an escape, and so prolonged narrow-objective focus can also cause chronic muscle pain.

While stress is unavoidable in life, it need not be a permanent state. Stress can be thought of as a force that squeezes our body and mind. And stress isn't necessarily a bad thing—it can help us get things done, take action, change, and grow. Stress is negative only when it's unrelenting and accumulating. While some stress naturally dissipates after an emergency, some of it lingers in our body in the form of tense muscles, constricted blood vessels, pressure on nerves, and other physical conditions.

Open-Focus training—learning to flexibly move out of narrow-objective attention—is a normalizing process, a way of reversing the clenching impact of stress and allowing all systems to return to equilibrium. By and large, the problems caused by stress are functional rather than structural, though if stress is left untreated, its effects can become structural.

In Open Focus, the sympathetic nervous system—which drives the body's fight-or-flight reactions—starts to quiet, and the parasympathetic system engages the body's slower, more relaxed functions, such as digestion. Blood flow returns again into the many parts of the body where function had been diminished, waking them up, healing them, improving their function, bringing them back online. Muscles, from our eye and face muscles to heart and lungs, enjoy increased blood flow and become less tense. The longer we dwell in this balanced, open-attention realm, the more stress the body is allowed to diffuse and the more healing can take place.

And in diffuse-immersed attention, stress is diffused as it arises, which means the process is self-balancing and stabilizing. In other words, we might still feel fearful in stressful situations, but rather than trapping the fear in our body, we feel fear in a state of diffuse-immersed attention and it diffuses, diminishes, and disappears.

When the brain moves out of narrow focus, it processes at a slower speed and also becomes more stable. It's interesting to consider the case of Neurontin, a drug created to treat epileptic seizures. Epilepsy is the product of a brain that is electrically unstable, and neurons that are easily recruited by the spread of low-frequency theta brain waves can cause the loss of consciousness. While Neurontin works well for seizures—because it stabilizes the brain and stops the spread of slow brain-wave activity—it is also used "off label" (to treat problems for which it has not yet been proved effective) for a host of other conditions, from panic attacks to migraines to obsessive-compulsive disorder and chronic pain. That's because all of these problems are in part products of an electrically unstable brain.

Jack Dreyfus, founder of an investment company called the Dreyfus Fund, suffered depression for years. It was relieved by a drug called phenytoin (its brand name is Dilantin). Within an hour of taking phenytoin, he wrote, his symptoms of depression were greatly relieved. Dreyfus was so impressed, he launched a medical foundation and a campaign to get the word out about the miracle drug. The drug was nearing the end of its patent, though, and Parke-Davis, the company that owned it, was reluctant to promote it. But it's been used to treat a host of seemingly unrelated problems, from anxiety to mood disorders, bed-wetting, migraines, arthritis, and even pain. Dilantin, like Neurontin, is a seizure medication that acts to stabilize runaway electrical activity in the brain.

A brain that is flexible—electrically stable most of the time and running at higher, more unstable speeds only when the situation dictates—is one that can deal with pain more effectively. Forty years of research and clinical observation show that Open-Focus exercises and training teach us to deploy our attention in a way that increases brain stability and flexibility.

The Four Styles of Attention

There is more to a healthy nervous system, though, than simply leaving behind the emergency aspects of narrow-objective focus and moving into the restfulness of diffuse and immersed attention. There are several other kinds of attention that we need to become aware of and utilize. The goal of Open-Focus training is not to favor or get stuck in any one attention style, but to make use of the full range and possible combinations of attention styles that are available simultaneously. Up to now in this book, the term *Open Focus* has been synonymous with diffuse, immersed attention and has been juxtaposed with narrow-objective attention. However, we can also think of Open Focus as an attention style that includes equal amounts of the four fundamental styles of attention: narrow, diffuse, objective, and immersed. The fact is, Open Focus also includes an awareness of how we are paying attention at any time, which allows us to select the appropriate style of attention for each situation.

I have identified four main types of attention: *diffuse, narrow, objective,* and *immersed* attention, all of which can occur more or less equally and simultaneously. You can be in narrow focus and diffuse focus simultaneously. Each fundamental style of attention is unique and, when it is emphasized, it has significant and different impacts on our physiology, moods, and behavior. Each of the physiological mechanisms that support the different kinds of attention are independent, which means the styles can—and do—exist simultaneously or in combination with the others.

In Open Focus all fundamental styles can exist simultaneously and equally. A flexible central nervous system is not biased toward the high arousal of narrow-objective focus or the low arousal of diffuse-immersed attention. Instead, the healthy nervous system naturally cycles through these styles. Along a spectrum, the central nervous system combines and supports a variety of attention styles around an alert and interested type of attention. In Open Focus, our attention is inclusive—sights, sounds, and other sensory information are all taken in, but in a broadly interested way, not in such a way that we focus on one sensory signal to the exclusion of all others.

Our attention, as I've said, in effect regulates our brain waves, and each of these different ways of attending causes a shift in the EEG (the graphic representation of the electrical activity of the brain as detected by sensors placed on the scalp). Brain-wave activity normally operates in the 1- to 40-hertz range. Delta (the slowest, from 0.5 to 4 hertz) is the sleep range. Theta (from 4 to 8 hertz) is the twilight of consciousness, between falling asleep and feeling deeply relaxed or daydreaming. Alpha (from 8 to 12 hertz) is also a relaxed state but one in which we are still alert and can function effectively. The active frequency, beta (from 13 to 40 hertz), is where we usually carry out our tasks and is usually divided into three categories: low, mid, and high range. Low beta (12 to 15 hertz) is characterized by relaxed but interested attention, typical of someone taking a test who knows the material well. Midrange beta (15 to 18 hertz) is focused external attention, and from here and above is associated with the exclusive use of narrow focus. High beta (18 hertz and higher) is correlated with tense muscles, anger, anxiety, and other intense emotions. Examples include someone taking an important test who doesn't know the material, or someone screaming with fright or anger at another driver because he was cut off.

Narrow Attention

Narrow attention, as I've mentioned, is the one style modern people favor the most, and our overuse of it causes many of our problems. It engages the brain's high frequencies, from mid to high beta, and is energetic and fast paced. It is an exclusive type of attention that addresses a limited subset of all available stimuli. Narrow attention focuses on a figure and apportions little or no awareness to the background or periphery. In its extreme, it approaches one-pointed attention.

Being aware of a human or another object separate from the landscape it appears on, and not including the landscape or other background, is narrow focus. Narrow attention isn't just about how we see. We can chronically narrow-focus on any sensation or thought or problem, to the exclusion of almost everything else. If we are having a conversation in narrow focus, for example, we might block out other sensory input, aside from the words being spoken and our private self-talk. As a result, our physical response to the content of the conversation might remain inaccessible to our attention.

On the other hand, if we are arguing with someone, we might narrow-focus on angry feelings and a sense of being wronged by the other person. In that case, the narrowness of our focus keeps us from listening to what the other person is saying, or makes it difficult for us to access thoughts and feelings that might end the fight.

We can listen intently for a certain sound and miss other sounds or the silence between them. Extreme narrow focus can be crippling when it is overused or chronic, bringing on anxiety, panic, worry, and a profound rigidity of focus. It is also the enemy of a smooth, fluid performance. A golfer, for example, who suffers what is known as the yips—uncontrollable muscle movements when putting—is hyperfocused, and his or her muscles are tense and spasming.

Objective Attention

Objective attention emotionally and perceptually distances the observer from the object of awareness and increases muscle tension. The combination of narrow focus and objective attention is energized and fast paced, favoring the rational and linear processing skills of the brain's left hemisphere. It emphasizes thinking and seeing while diminishing the role of the other senses, including emotions, and keeps the observer apart from the object of the attention. Rodin's sculpture *The Thinker* captures the posture of objective attention. The man is narrowly focused, either engaged with or separate from his thoughts. Objective attention has allowed humans to step back from union with the natural world. This helped our early ancestors in the discovery of the laws of nature and to develop science and technology.

Immersed Attention

Immersed, or absorbed, attention is more pronounced in the theta and low-alpha realms, and is characteristic of people who enter into union with an object or activity and forget themselves. This kind of unselfconsciousness can be pleasurable. The effortlessness of a performing artist or an athlete is well learned. A dancer so

95

immersed in her body, movement, and music that she loses a sense of self or where she is, for example, exhibits immersed attention. Both diffuse and immersed attention appear to involve the right hemisphere of the brain.

There is also a combination of *narrow and immersed* attention, which is associated with a combination of low and high brain-wave frequencies occurring simultaneously. Immersed awareness is a way of attending that allows us to savor and intensify an experience. Narrow-immersed attention includes intellectually interesting or emotionally and physically pleasant and stimulating activities—any experience we want to move physically closer to, in order to intensify and savor the experience. Part of the attraction of a sporting event or symphony is the ability to become absorbed or immersed with minimum self-consciousness.

Diffuse Attention

Diffuse attention is just what it sounds like—a softer, less focused, more inclusive view of the world. In diffuse attention, we're not attending to any one thing but opening to everything, equally and simultaneously. This form of attention may emphasize a figure on a landscape, but there is a simultaneous awareness of the equal importance of the ground, the landscape around the figure, as well as the ground of experience, space.

Diffuse attention is panoramic, rather than single-pointed, and in its most extreme form is all-inclusive, three-dimensional, and gives equal and simultaneous attention to all internal and external stimuli and the space in which they occur. It supports multisensory experience, not just thinking and seeing, which are the senses that dominate in narrow focus. Walking through a meadow and being simultaneously aware of the sound of birds singing, the smell of flowers, the feel of a breeze, the view of the trees, and the space and the silence in which these sensory experiences occur, is diffuse focus.

The inclusion of narrow and diffuse attention in a balanced way is appropriate for most of the things we encounter day to day. While narrow focus concentrates and intensifies awareness, diffuse focus spreads and moderates both the experience and our reactions to it.

Emerging from Narrow Focus

Learning to open your focus is like cracking open the door to a dark room. Opening it a crack allows enough light so that many of the objects in the dark can be seen. Some air may enter the room, making it easier to breathe. Opening the door even a crack can change our perceptual and physical environment in a big way.

While all of the four ways of attending discussed in this chapter are indeed part of everyone's biological equipment—though genetics, I believe, determine the robustness of their impact—few of us can look up from this book and instantly see, for example, the living room wall, paintings, and furniture in diffuse focus. Moving out of narrow focus is like unclenching a fist that has been clenched for years. After a life lived in chronic narrow-objective focus, we are too habituated to break out of it easily. Emerging from narrow focus is not about just taking in peripheral awareness, but infusing all objects and space with an equal and simultaneous awareness. It's a skill that takes time to learn. With some specialized exercises, however, anyone can learn to change the way he or she pays attention.

Being able to flexibly deploy your attention can relieve your pain right away, and it can help you feel and localize it, which is a good first step toward dissolving pain and living a pain-free life. Sometimes we repress pain successfully. We don't feel it, or we feel it as tension, though the pain is there, along with our resistance to it, taking a toll. Any pain, emotional or physical, has a feeling associated with it in the body. Once you feel it, you can dissolve it, and I suggest how to do that in the next chapter.

Mary, a client of mine, noticed a real shift when she started Open-Focus training. She benefited even more when she started the next level of training, in which she learned to dissolve her migraine headaches. "The first time I tried the dissolving pain technique, it was a real turning point right away, almost magical," she said. "I realized that I didn't have to live with the pain and that I had it in myself to get rid of it. It was really a revelation."

By the time she stopped coming to the clinic, she was having one severe headache a month and was looking forward to eliminating that. She felt empowered, she said, to know that she was in control. "I feel better knowing I have some role in making pain go away," she said. "You feel the world is a better place."

Open-Focus training helped more than just her migraines. In her job with a public relations firm, she writes a lot. "My writing flows more easily when I sit down to write, and the results are a lot better," she said. "I don't have writer's block." Open Focus also helped her running. "I'll be running along and I'll start to feel a little head pain as I am running, and by melting into those feelings, it becomes much less effortful and I perform better. Runners talk of peak experience. Through Open Focus, you can make that happen. You can be in touch with the moment and be in touch with your body."

8

Dissolving Pain

Each of us literally chooses, by his way of attending to things, what sort of universe he should appear to himself to inhabit.

—WILLIAM JAMES

MARY ANNE HAD the pain and other symptoms of multiple sclerosis when she came to see us, including foot drop (weakness in the front lower legs, foot, ankle, and toes), muscle tremors, and leg drag. MS is an autoimmune disorder in which the body's immune system attacks the myelin sheaths (the casing that surrounds nerve fibers), causing them to deteriorate. Nerve fibers transmit electrical impulses within the brain and between the brain and spinal cord and the rest of the body, including the muscles and organs. As the sheaths break down, they harden into a type of scar tissue, and the messages between the nervous system and the body go awry, causing, among other things, motor problems.

Open-Focus training cannot repair the deterioration of the myelin sheaths; that's a breakdown in the body's structure. Instead, Mary Anne came to see us for the stress and anxiety she suffered, caused by her concern about her symptoms and other issues. As she worked with the Open-Focus exercises and learned to dissolve the pain in her legs and elsewhere, she began to notice that her other symptoms started to diminish. The foot drop and leg drag, for example, occurred much less, and her tremors were often only barely noticeable.

"Sometimes I have the symptoms, and sometimes I don't have them at all," she told me one day, very pleased. Over time, she found that she was able to live in Open Focus and stay pain-free. She adds, "I used to have to say to myself, 'Open your focus, diffuse your attention,' but now it's reflexive, and it's very much a part of me."

Learning to Merge Awareness and Pain

Have you ever carried a heavy suitcase for a couple of blocks? You might notice that while you carry the bag, your arms, shoulder, and neck are strained, but you really feel the pain after you set the suitcase down. It's similar to what happens with Open Focus.

We all carry tension and pain in our muscles and throughout our body, but we often don't feel that tension and pain in our day-to-day life, keeping it successfully submerged below a conscious level. One of the reasons we are so attached to narrow-objective focus is that it successfully represses the pain, at least in the short run. And we would keep directing our attention away from our pain, if it didn't eventually surface into conscious awareness.

Once we move into diffuse focus, though, we crack the shell around the pain, breaking the narrow-objective-attention loop, and we start to feel the pain, which is a necessary step in dissolving it. It might not surface as pain per se, but as tension or one of many other kinds of feelings, from muscle tremors to tingling sensations, waves of pleasure, or emotionally charged memories.

As I mentioned, sometimes moving into diffuse attention is enough for pain to simply rise up, be experienced, and dissolve on its own. Think of a cold piece of toast with a pat of butter on it. The toast is you; the butter is your pain. Cold toast is you in narrow-objective focus. As you start to move into a diffuse style of attention, you (the toast) warm, and the pain (the butter) dissolves into the bread. When you move into a more diffuse attention, you are becoming warmer, and your muscles are softer, more able to admit the pain and let it diffuse. That's what happened with Michael and his migraines.

Sometimes, however, the pain is more stubborn, or our resistance to it is greater. At this point, we need to do the opposite of what our instincts usually tell us to do. In response to pain, our habit is to distance ourselves from the pain and to fight it, thinking that if we don't resist the pain, it will intensify. *But over the long term, exactly the reverse is true. We exacerbate the pain by narrow-focusing away from it or otherwise trying to resist it, consciously or unconsciously. After we open our attention into a diffuse awareness, we need to learn to move toward the pain, allowing it to melt into a broadened awareness, and so let it dissolve.* That's what Mary was able to do on a continuing basis, as symptoms arose. There is almost no feeling we cannot heal or mitigate in this way. I've had clients tell me that they have bruised a shin and been able to heal it more quickly by melting into the pain, or reduce the symptoms of a cold or flu, or speed the healing of a cut.

To dissolve pain, it's important to experience pain in the realm of feeling. You can visualize the pain, and that might help some, but the best effect will come from being able to feel the pain fully.

Putting Pain in a Larger Context

The reason the intensity of pain is amplified by narrow-objective focus is not because the pain itself physiologically increases, but because the pain fills the constricted scope of our narrow attention. Narrow-objective attention causes our pain to become a much bigger deal than it really is because it fills our entire constricted awareness rather than being only a fraction of our broadened awareness.

Walk up to a brick wall and look at a single brick. That lone brick is all you see and think about, because it occupies your entire awareness. Back off a little bit and the brick becomes one in a wall of many. Move a little farther away and the brick wall becomes part of a home. Move still farther away and the home is one in a neighborhood. Farther yet and the neighborhood is part of a city. And as you move even farther, the city is part of a state and the country and the earth circling the sun.

When we allow a diffuse-immersed attention to grow around a narrow-objective attention on pain, physiological arousal levels are lowered. There's a saying, "Don't sweat the small stuff." In a broadened, diffuse awareness, we have gained context, a view of the big picture—and all pain is small stuff, no big deal. Accepting the pain and then moving even closer to it, absorbing and diffusing it in our awareness, becomes much easier.

Why does how we attend affect painful muscles? As I mentioned earlier, in fight-or-flight mode, muscles are tense. Emergency function constricts blood vessels and redirects blood flow to certain areas of the body needed for quick and powerful action. This reduces the oxygen available to other muscles and nerves. As we open our focus, both in general and around the injured area, there is a robust physiological change. Expanding awareness around a specific site brings blood to that site, increases circulation in the vessels and nerves, and promotes site-specific healing. That is why dissolving pain can prevent swelling and inflammation and can allow for more rapid healing, reduce or eliminate bruises, and relax muscles in spasm.

I can't quite say, "I've never met a pain that can't be dissolved through the use of attention skills." I can almost say it because even pain that is mostly physical or structural—for example, from surgery or a wound—can be dissolved. There are people who aren't good at using attention skills or don't stay with their use, but virtually any kind of pain I have worked with has dissolved in this way. I can think of only a relative few exceptions in the nearly forty years I've used attention skills in the treatment of pain.

Take the case of Maryanne, one of my colleagues. She had first seen me after surgery for a plantar wart on her foot. The incision where the wart was removed wouldn't close. After several sessions, the hole closed and the incision healed.

But the real test for Maryanne came after she underwent bowel surgery. One of the common aftereffects of the type of surgery she had is adhesions, or fibrous scar tissue that forms in and around the site of the incision. They can be extraordinarily painful and often get worse with time. Maryanne had taught Open-Focus workshops and knew the techniques well. She could gain some relief using the techniques on her own. But the pain was so severe she wasn't able to stay with it as long as she needed to in order to get relief. She called and I agreed to guide her to dissolve her pain over the phone. Sometimes, in the case of persistent, severe pain, having someone coach you can bring better results.

During the first few sessions, the pain was very intrusive, and it took twenty-five minutes to dissolve the pain from 10 to 0, the point at which she didn't feel any pain. Over the next few treatments, it took less time to dissolve her pain, until it was down to ten minutes, and with each session the effects lasted longer. Now when Maryanne does a dissolving pain session on her own, the pain dissolves and stays gone for as long as three days. "By the time the exercises were done," she said, "I was able to completely merge my awareness into the pain; I was able to spread my pain over my entire body, and finally spread it through my skin and outside of my skin to the space outside of my body until every vestige of pain was dissolved."

Merging with Pain—and Other Techniques for Dissolving It

Learning to dissolve pain begins by moving into the physically quiet, low-frequency styles of attention. Some practitioners can shift instantly into Open Focus, while others may need to listen to a half-hour-long exercise. In any case, after clients localize their pain, and the space in and around it, they imagine moving toward it and letting the pain spread throughout their awareness, and letting their awareness spread through their pain. Others may prefer bathing in it. In either case, the pain is no longer held only in the center of attention as an object, at a distance, in narrow-objective attention, but we have opened the scope of our awareness and have merged with the pain. As I mentioned earlier, it's the same thing we do with pleasurable feelings—let them in and then they naturally dissolve.

There are several different techniques for dissolving pain. It's possible to learn to narrow-focus on the precise location of pain and consciously dive into the heart of it, as I did with kidney-stone pain. It's like diving into a swimming pool when you know the water is cold, but you do it anyway. It's faster, but not everyone can or is willing to do it. Some clients need to take more time to work their way gradually toward the pain's location and dissolution. Still others prefer to passively allow the pain to migrate toward them until it merges with them.

Another generally successful method is broadly diffusing one's attention around the center of the localized pain. This method allows the pain to spread, expand, and dissipate through its surroundings to the point of dissolution.

Another form of attention is simply diffusing attention and doing that sufficiently in stages, more and more broadly, until the pain is released into the background of Open-Focus awareness.

Another technique is the opposite: it involves locating the pain within the body. Feel the region in which the pain is harbored (anxiety might be experienced in the back of the head or stomach, for example). Feel the pain in the body while at the same time feeling the whole body around it. Then feel into this area of the chest or stomach or head or wherever the pain is, and feel for the boundaries or shape of the pain and the space around those boundaries and the space that the shape occupies. Then find the smaller region within that pain where it is most intense. Continue to repeat the process of feeling for the strongest spot within the existing shape of the pain until the pain disappears. On a physical level, each time we do this, we are bringing more blood to the site of the pain.

Working with Multiple Pains Simultaneously

Even if more than one type of pain is present, they can all be dissolved, serially or simultaneously. We might have neck pain, for example, and also an intense headache. It's best to dissolve the highest-intensity pain first because it's usually easier to pay attention to it and it would constitute a significant distraction otherwise. And sometimes pains, even though seemingly separate in the body, are connected. With practice, multiple pains can be dissolved simultaneously.

A fear of feeling pain or its increase in intensity often accompanies physical pain and becomes part of the problem. In this case, it can help to dissolve the fear or resistance to experiencing the feeling. Some people, as odd as this might sound, also fear the loss of their pain. They may have lived with it for so many years that it has become part of their identity. They don't know who they would be without the pain, so they fear losing it. This fear can and needs to be dissolved as well.

It's critical not to try too hard to dissolve the pain. Trying hard creates tension, and tension creates or eventually exacerbates pain. You don't have to strain and reach for the pain; it's already there. Just allow the pain in and let this awareness, which is you, become wholly vulnerable to the pain, and let it spread, diffuse, and dissolve.

Notice how the exercise questions ask whether you can *imagine* feeling the space, not whether you *can* feel the space. This choice of words is important in promoting the sense of effortlessness that's needed. Chronic repression of pain causes an immense energy drain, and once pain has been dissolved, energy is liberated. Remember that feeling of clarity and lightness that appeared after I dissolved my kidney pain? Clients who have treated their pain with Open-Focus skills often feel more centered, as if they have slipped back into their own "skin" after a long absence.

Where Does the Pain Go?

Where does the pain go when we diffuse it? What is happening in the brain in this model?

Our brain has two notable body maps represented in it: a sensory map in the somatosensory cortex and a motor map in the frontal cortex. Moving to diffuse and immersed attention encourages phase-synchronous alpha, the powerful healing brain-wave rhythm. Pain, meanwhile, is narrowly objectified in higher-frequency asynchronous activity. When our attention is diffused and immersed, most of the brain is engaged in phase-synchronous activity. So as we move into diffuse focus and the brain becomes synchronous, the asynchronous pain rhythms are also recruited and gradually become more synchronous, and if attention is diffused and immersed long enough and completely enough, the pain is no longer narrowly objectified and disappears. What happens to the pain in the brain is not unlike a puff of smoke that starts out thick and visible and then slowly diffuses, spreads out, and dissipates into the air until it can no longer be seen.

During some exercises, I'll ask a client to bring the pain back into awareness. When that happens, it's very clear how we are all involved in creating the experience of pain. Then I'll ask the client to dissolve it, and the pain diffuses into the space from which it arose. That is, pain diffuses and becomes part of the all-around attention we call diffuse-immersed attention. Learning to create the experience of pain, then make it disappear, and then make it reappear again, is good practice for learning flexibility of attention.

Another way to think about this phenomenon is that when we objectify, as we do with pain, we create a sense of self, a sense of being separate from the world around us. And the existence of the self is what it takes to experience pain. When the usual sense of self disappears—as it does in Open Focus—the asynchronous activity in the brain disappears, and there is no interference pattern or "self" to experience pain.

Remember that it's not only physical pain that you are learning to dissolve with these exercises but any unwanted experience. While you are engaging in a dissolving pain exercise, for example, you might be distracted by the ringing of a telephone or the beeping of a car horn or the tingling of an itch. Rather than fighting the urge to respond—which is what we do in narrow focus—you can approach the distraction as if it were a pain. Let your awareness broaden to encompass the distraction and then merge with it and include it in your experience so it can be alleviated.

With training and practice, dissolving pain becomes second nature. In the same way that working a muscle makes it stronger and better able to carry out its tasks, as we learn to live a life in Open Focus, we become more adept at dissolving pain and other unwanted experiences as they arise, ideally without even thinking about it.

Exercise

Dissolving Pain

This exercise helps you to dissolve any pain present in your body. A beginner to this process may benefit by listening to the General Training exercise first, followed immediately by this Dissolving Pain exercise (which can be found on tracks 2 and 3, respectively, on the enclosed audio CD). After some practice with general training, one may go directly to the dissolving pain exercise.

When pain is absent consider using this exercise for dissolving the pressure of the chair upon your body, a sense of gravity, or a sense of self.

For information on downloading a recording of this exercise, please see page 183.

If you are reading this exercise aloud, remember to allow fifteen seconds between the end of one question and the beginning of the next question.

Guiding Questions

Can you imagine adopting a gently correct posture and moving as little as possible with your eyes closed?

Can you imagine feeling the space that the whole room occupies?

Can you imagine feeling the space that your whole body occupies?

Is it possible for you to imagine feeling the space of the whole room you are in and the space your entire body occupies simultaneously?

Is it possible for you to imagine that as you inhale naturally, your breath fills the entire volume of your body?

And can you imagine that as you exhale naturally and as your breath leaves your body, your body is left occupied by space?

At the same time you're aware of the space your body occupies, is it possible for you to imagine the space on all sides of your body simultaneously?

At the same time you're aware of the space inside and the space outside of your body, can you imagine feeling the volume of any pain or discomfort you may experience?

Is it possible for you to imagine the length, width, and thickness—the dimensions and shape—of any pain or discomfort you may feel?

Can you imagine feeling the space between the center of the pain or discomfort you feel and the back of your body?

Can you imagine feeling the space between the center of your pain and the sides of your body? Can you imagine feeling the space between the center of your pain and the front of your body?

Is it possible for you to imagine feeling the space between the center of your pain and the top of your head?

Can you imagine feeling the space between your pain and the space inside your ears?

Can you imagine feeling the space between your pain and the space inside your mouth and cheeks?

Can you imagine feeling the space between your pain and the space inside your throat?

Is it possible for you to imagine feeling the space between your pain and the space inside your stomach?

Can you imagine feeling the space between your pain and the space inside your lower trunk, midsection, upper trunk, neck, head, limbs, digits, and internal organs?

Is it possible for you to imagine feeling the space between your pain and the closest part of your spine?

Is it possible for you to imagine that as you inhale naturally, your breath flows through the heart of your pain?

Can you imagine that as you exhale naturally, your breath flows through the heart of your pain?

Is it possible for you to imagine that you neither reject nor encourage the feeling of pain?

Can you imagine fully accepting the feeling presence of your pain but neither encouraging nor avoiding it in any way?

Can you imagine allowing your pain to diffuse in any direction and through any region of your body where it may naturally and effortlessly go?

Is it possible for you to imagine feeling the surface area of your entire body and at the same time remain open to the feeling of your pain in the center of your awareness?

Can you imagine feeling that the boundaries of your body are gradually dissolving, so that the space inside and the space outside of your body become continuous? And at the same time, can you imagine that the boundaries of your pain are also dissolving, allowing your pain to spread in every direction?

At the same time you're aware of your feeling of pain, is it possible for you also to attend equally to any other sensations and perceptions that are available—tastes, smells, thoughts, images, sounds, body feelings, or emotions—attending equally and simultaneously to these sensations and to the three-dimensional space in which they exist?

Can you imagine that this three-dimensional space permeates and pervades all of your sensations and perceptions, and your pain?

Can you imagine gently narrowing your attention and centering it upon the pain that you experience?

Can you imagine that this awareness, which is you, can intermingle with the pain, at the body location where you perceive the pain to be, gently, effortlessly moving through the pain and also letting the pain spread through you?

As awareness and pain intermingle, is it possible for you to imagine that this awareness, which is you, can dissolve right into the pain—and the pain can permeate your awareness—each remaining vulnerable to space?

As you reach the heart of the pain—that part of the pain that is most intense, the center of the pain—can you imagine gradually opening your awareness once again and allowing the pain to spread into and through the center of your awareness and experiencing all of the other sensations and perceptions that are available to you, to be attended to equally and simultaneously in three-dimensional space?

Can you imagine that in Open-Focus attention, there needn't be any movement?

Can you imagine that Open Focus is an effortless process of attention in which you can rest and function as well?

Is it possible for you to narrow your attention, and as you direct it toward your pain, is it possible for you to imagine that you can open yourself to the experience of pain more subtly and more completely as you approach it? And can you imagine allowing the pain to spread through this awareness-space, which is you?

And can you imagine that as you begin to enter the pain, you even more completely open yourself, making yourself more vulnerable to the experience of pain, surrendering yourself right into the heart, the center of the pain? And just as you experience the most intense part of the pain, can you imagine once again letting the pain spread through you and your body and space and opening your attention to include all that is you—all attention styles, sensations, perceptions, emotions, and feelings, including the pain—all simultaneously and equally and once again coming to rest in multisensory space?

Once again, can you imagine guiding your attention toward your pain? And at the same time, can you imagine moving toward the pain and opening yourself more completely and more totally to the full experience of whatever pain you may encounter, surrendering yourself finally into the heart essence of the pain until, just as you experience the maximum pain, you once again let your pain spread through your open attention, your Open Focus, to include also all other sensations and perceptions that are present, coming to rest once again in Open Focus?

Can you imagine repeating this cycle, starting in an Open Focus permeated by three-dimensional and multisensory space and narrowing your attention and directing it toward the pain, and moving toward the pain and fully experiencing all of your pain until you have experienced the most intense part of your pain, letting the pain spread through awareness-space and returning to Open-Focus attention?

Can you imagine repeating this cycle at your own pace until your pain dissolves completely?

9

Eye, Head, and Neck Tension and Pain

Pain is inevitable. Suffering is optional.
—Anonymous

After consulting many doctors, Marie came to my clinic to see if I could help with the painful ringing in her ears called tinnitus. Tinnitus is a noise that occurs for no apparent reason, and can be extremely painful, distracting, and disabling. Some describe the sound variously as a clanging or a squeal or a screech. A character in Thomas Hardy's novel *A Pair of Blue Eyes* describes his tinnitus as the sound of frying: "People frying fish: fry, fry, fry all day long in my poor head." Tinnitus can keep people from working and from enjoying their lives, and some people are driven to near madness because of the sound. There are several different types of tinnitus with different causes. There are some types that respond very well to Open-Focus training, and Marie's was one of those.

Marie started with Head and Hands two or three times a day at home. Part of the reason for that is that Head and Hands helps reduce anxiety and stress, which often accompany tinnitus. Open-Focus training also started to open her awareness to the top of her jaw (in the vicinity of the temporomandibular joint), to the point where she could feel tension, discomfort, and pain in the muscles there, feelings she had repressed. A lot of the clients I see with tense and clenched muscles often are not aware they are clenched because they have been that way for so long and they have shut down all feeling. It's not uncommon for someone to have tense muscles throughout his or her body but not know it and even claim to feel relaxed. This was my own case.

In the Open-Focus approach, the ability to feel tension and pain is a good thing. It's the first step toward being able to dissolve the discomfort. As soreness in her jaw muscles started to surface, Marie brought the dissolving pain exercises into play, repeatedly moving her attention toward the pain and tension. The more she could feel the discomfort, the easier it became to dissolve. After six or seven sessions, the tension in the muscles was released. As muscle elasticity returned, the ringing in her ears diminished and then ceased altogether.

My theory about this type of tinnitus is that tight muscles in the neck and around the ear make the parts of the middle and inner ear taut, especially the stapedius muscles, which attach to the ossicles and modulate transmission of sound in the middle and inner ear. The ossicles vibrate because they are so taut. A combination of factors may increase stress and tension—a loud sound or an unpleasant emotional event. These may set off tinnitus in the compromised ear. Sometimes, if muscle tension does not seem to be the problem, I've asked people with tinnitus to dissolve the sound they are hearing in the same way as I would with a pain, and this tends to work quite well.

The head and neck are singled out for special treatment in this chapter because so many people have problems in these regions, whether it be migraines or cluster headaches, torticollis (wryneck), chronic neck pain, stiffness or rigidity, jaw pain, teeth grinding, eye tension or vision problems, or several of these things combined. It's understandable because much of the way we use our head and neck causes muscle tension. Holding our head up as we watch computer monitors or driving in traffic for long, stressful periods strains the head, neck, and eyes. The shoulders, too, are involved in this, and tension there can affect much of the head, face, and neck. Even simple movements often involve the overuse of the eyes, jaw, neck, shoulders, and other muscles necessary to accomplish the action. When shoulder muscles are contracted, the neck, head, and face can be drawn down. A typist who looks at the keyboard, for example, rather than the monitor, might stress the neck and shoulders and also depress his breathing. And it's likely that we are genetically predisposed to respond to stress in an idiosyncratic pattern over the course of our lives.

Emotional stress activates the muscles of the head and neck as well. Bracing ourselves in response to any kind of threatening situation tenses these muscles. After the threat is gone, the muscles can remain tense in spite of the fact that we feel we are at rest. More so than other parts of the body, the head, neck, shoulders, and trapezius muscles are prone to stress problems. These are the alertness or vigilance muscles, which are vital to making our way in the world, being hyperalert to assure our safety, and responding to perceived danger with emergency reactions.

Eye muscles are among the parts of the body that are most sensitive to emotional stress. They are responsible for seeing and perceiving things around us that might threaten our well-being, and these concerns lead us to chronically narrow our focus of attention and tighten eye and face muscles. This distorts the eyeball, restricts its movement, and affects vision.

The muscles of our eyes, like the rest of our physiology, are far more flexible than we assume, which means they can be tense and their movement restricted because of stress, physical and emotional.

Emotional factors might, in fact, make the greatest changes in our vision, and they can also lead to learning disabilities. I know of a young man who had grown up in a chaotic environment. As he came home from school every day, he grew nervous and fearful, worried that his abusive and alcoholic father would beat him again.

The young man ended up in a school for children who had been traumatized, and his teachers noticed that he had trouble reading and writing. Among other things, abuse and neglect at an early age often affect a child's cognitive abilities. In this case, the young man's eyes had been affected by trauma. The problem wasn't that he needed glasses. The emotional stress had caused his field of vision to become so narrow that he could see only one word at a time. Teachers at the school taught him to relax his eye muscles, and eventually, as his visual scope grew broader, he could see one, two, and three words at a time, and finally phrases. Just like the nervous system, the eye is plastic, or changeable, and can be brought back into function.

Our ability to change the functioning of our eyes is well demonstrated in the story of the "sea gypsies." Swedish researcher Anna Gislén, of Lund University, went to Thailand to investigate a group of indigenous people called the Mokken who live on boats or houses on stilts and dive for seafood. The Mokken's young children are trained to collect edible sea creatures ten to fifteen feet down on the ocean floor, where they can tell stones from clams without diving masks or other visual aids. Gislén's study, published in *Current Biology* in 2003, found that the children have learned to change the shape of their lenses to increase refraction and allow them to see at such depths. They are also able to constrict their pupils to help them see clearly.

At first it was thought these children's visual abilities might be a genetic adaptation to their environment, since European children, who do not have the same need to forage for food at the bottom of the sea, don't seem to have these abilities. But in fairly short order, Lund was able to teach Swedish children to gain similar control over their eye muscles and lenses.

We can all learn to gain some control over our eye muscles. They are often distorted from a healthy state by a lifetime of stress, and with Open-Focus training, we can restore them to their natural flexibility. Releasing tension in the eyes can greatly improve our vision. ·

The selection and control of images falling on the eye is carried out by three extremely fine and distinct muscle systems. One system is located on the outside of the eyeball, and the other two inside the eye. The iris is an inside muscle, which regulates the amount of light entering the eye by varying pupil diameter. The ciliary body, a ring of muscle around the lens, is an internal muscle system that adjusts the shape of the lens to bring near and far objects into focus. The third set of muscles, attached to the sclera, or outside covering of the eye, is responsible for tracking and pointing the eye in various directions to scan and search.

Our eyes are also changed by physical stress because of how we use them in modern life. Before the industrial revolution, humans paid attention in very different ways, working outdoors on a variety of tasks. And in the days of hunters and gatherers, people varied their attention—looking up from their handwork to see expansive views, scanning the horizon for the movement of game, for example. With the advent of writing and the dominance of the written word, reading began to restrict our visual aperture for long periods of time. As people migrated to assembly lines in factories or to office cubicles, how we see and pay attention began to change dramatically for much of the day.

Prolonged close-in focusing now dominates much of our normal day. Working at computers, reading technical documents, or performing a repetitive task on a factory assembly line can cause serious eyestrain. Moreover, eye muscles are both voluntary and involuntary, and forcing ourselves to pay attention to things we need to see, rather than letting our desire to see control visual function, causes even more eyestrain.

The number of things that require attention has grown dramatically, and trying to make sense of it all is demanding. One issue of the Sunday *New York Times* contains more information than all of the material available to readers in the fifteenth century. Sixty thousand books are published in the United States each year, and there are more than two billion pages on the Internet.

We also live in an object-oriented society, and we find ourselves awash in a sea of visual images and sense objects. Stores are crammed with thousands of things; more and more objects are featured in television, print, and online ads. On a daily basis, we are shown an array of material items that would simply have astounded people of earlier eras.

In the midst of this visual onslaught, our default mode of attending is narrow-objective focus, which we use to wade through this torrent and quickly classify what is important and what is not. It requires a great deal of energy to take it all in and sort it out. Too often, our narrow, rigid attention to the world around us creates the fatigue of rigid attention syndrome (RAS), which is a source of many health problems.

In addition to more eyestrain, there are many other muscles in the head, neck, and trapezius that tense and strain to support narrow-objective attention, which in turn leads to everything from headaches to neck pain, other kinds of discomfort, and tension pains.

The Open-Focus approach can be directed to different regions of the body. And while general Open-Focus practices can help vision, imagining space in and around the eye brings about the release of tension in these specific muscle areas, and clients report that long-term vision problems such as nearsightedness improve, sometimes dramatically. Releasing muscles of the forehead, neck, and face, which support narrow-objective attention, can also help vision problems.

It's not only our vision that is affected by chronic narrow focus. Our stressed eyes can also contribute to vertigo. Jim, for example, was a client who suffered chronic dizziness and blurred vision, a problem that had gone on for years. After visits with doctors and specialists and rounds of medication, he came to our clinic. A couple of sessions of Open Focus caused tension and pain to surface at the back of his eyes, a place where people commonly hold tension. During the next session, he moved toward those feelings in a diffuse style of attention, dissolving them, bringing both his blurred vision and his dizziness to an end.

There's almost no end to the effects of stress on the eyes, and there are few such symptoms Open-Focus training cannot help. My wife, Susan, had dry eye syndrome. It is a painful and very uncomfortable problem, and the only treatment she knew of was inserting eyedrops every twenty minutes or so. Six years after this difficulty began, Susan started using Open-Focus exercises for her eyes, which guided her in becoming aware of space inside, outside, and around her eyes and head. After a month of using the "Eye-Centered Open Focus" exercise, her eyes started feeling better, and she was able to discontinue using the eyedrops except at bedtime. Not only did her dry eye condition get better, but her vision went from twenty-fifty to twenty-twenty.

We have witnessed a number of vision improvements consonant with Open-Focus training. The most dramatic improvement was in a young single mother who exhibited 20/200 vision (legally blind) at the onset of training and 20/20 at the end.

Exercise

Eye-Centered Open Focus

If you have a history of problems with your vision or your eyes themselves, but no symptoms are currently present, you can use this exercise intermittently, as a preventative measure. If your symptoms are present, use this exercise regularly. (See your physician to rule out medical problems.)

Remember to allow fifteen seconds between the end of one question and the beginning of the next question, and to close your eyes during these exercises early in training.

Guiding Questions

Can you imagine sitting gently upright and balancing yourself over your hips, with your eyes closed?

Can you imagine that your imagination happens freely and effortlessly?

Can you imagine that volume and distance are experienced the same way as space, like the sense of absence between your fingers, like the space your fingers occupy?

Can you imagine centering your foreground attention upon feeling, and especially upon the feeling of space, while including other sense experiences and their space in the surround or background of your attention?

Can you imagine centering your attention upon the sense of space surrounding and penetrating through feeling sensations?

Can you imagine that initially you may be able to narrow-focus upon the feeling of one body space at a time as the body spaces are mentioned in this exercise?

Can you imagine that with continued practice, your attention will broaden so that you will become able to add together your separate experiences of individual body spaces into a feeling of one whole space?

Can you imagine what it would feel like if you were already feeling the presence of your whole body while feeling the space your body occupies and the space around and through the boundaries of your body?

Can you imagine what it would feel like if you were already feeling the presence of your eyes and the space they occupy and the space around and through your eyes?

Can you imagine feeling the location of your eyes within the space your body occupies?

Can you imagine what it would be like to feel the space between your eyes and your breastbone?

Can you imagine feeling the space between your eyes and your backbone?

Is it possible for you to imagine feeling the space between your eyes and your throat and mouth?

Can you imagine feeling the space between your eyes and the space inside your stomach?

Can you imagine feeling the space between your eyes and each of your ribs on both sides of your chest?

Is it possible for you to imagine what it would be like to feel the distance between your eyes and the space inside your nose, your sinuses, your throat, your windpipe, and your lungs?

Can you imagine feeling the distance between your eyes and the space inside your mouth, your throat, your stomach, and your lower digestive system?

Can you imagine the space between your eyes and your waist?

Can you imagine the space between your eyes and the region between your navel and your backbone?

Can you imagine what it would be like to feel the space between your eyes and the region between your middle and lower spine?

Can you imagine the space between your eyes and the region between your hips?

Is it possible for you to imagine the space between your eyes and your buttocks, upper legs, knees, lower legs, ankles, feet, and toes?

Can you imagine feeling the space between your eyes and the region under your arms?

Can you imagine the space between your eyes and your shoulders, upper arms, elbows, wrists, hands, and fingers?

Can you imagine what it would feel like to experience the space around and permeating your eyes and the space around and permeating the soles of your feet and the palms of your hands—all simultaneously?

Can you imagine what it would feel like to experience the space between your eyes and your shoulder blades?

Can you imagine the space between your eyes and your lips, tongue, teeth, gums, and the space inside your mouth and cheeks?

Can you imagine the space between your eyes and the space between your cheeks?

Can you imagine the space between your eyes and your jaw?

Can you imagine the space between your eyes and the space inside your ears and the space between your ears?

Can you imagine the space between your eyes and the region of space inside and between your temples?

Can you imagine the space between your eyes and your eyelids, your eyebrows, and your forehead?

Can you imagine the space between your eyes and the back of your head and the top of your head and the sides of your head?

Can you imagine the space between your eyes and your whole head and face?

Can you imagine the space between your eyes and the still air touching your skin all over your body?

Can you imagine what it would be like to feel the sense of presence of your eyes as clouds of atoms floating in space— a space that extends in every direction and as far as you can imagine?

Is it possible for you to imagine what it would feel like to experience the space around your eyes and the space continuous and permeating through the cloud of atoms that is your heart?

Can you imagine feeling the space between the location of the feeling awareness that is you and the location of your eyes?

Can you imagine the cloud of feeling awareness and the clouds of atoms that are your eyes, floating toward each other and becoming one feeling experience, one combined cloud of awareness and eyes?

Is it possible for you to imagine that any emotions or other body feelings that are currently present are also experienced as clouds of feeling floating in space?

Can you imagine now that these clouds of emotion and other feelings also intermingle with the clouds of your awareness, floating in space?

Is it possible for you now to imagine the space that permeates each of your other senses: visualizing, hearing, tasting, smelling, thinking, and a sense of time?

Can you imagine that these clouds of sensation also merge with the clouds of awareness?

Can you imagine opening your eyes and also including seeing within your overall attention, without interfering in any way with your Open-Focus attention?

Can you now open your eyes and imagine seeing through objects and space, including your present visual experience, into your feeling-centered Open-Focus attention?

Can you imagine what it would be like for space to permeate your body-centered multisensory attention?

Can you imagine engaging in your daily activities while remaining centered in your body feeling?

Can you imagine paying attention to all sensation that is available to you, effortlessly and simultaneously surrounded and permeated by space?

Can you imagine practicing this exercise at least twice daily?

10

Emotions and Pain

We must embrace pain and use it as fuel for our journey.
—Poet Kenji Miyazawa

Janie had already been experiencing depression and anxiety when she was involved in a serious automobile accident. The top of a semitrailer she was driving behind snagged power lines, which pulled a telephone pole down and onto her car, crushing the top. The truck driver who caused the accident sped away and left her lying there for over an hour before she was found.

The accident and the physical pain from the collision accelerated her downward emotional spiral, and she was in great despair about her bad luck at having been in an accident, which in turn aggravated her tension and anxiety. Lethargic, unhappy, and in chronic pain, she had lain around the house, unable to motivate herself to get up and do anything. Pain medication and several antidepressant medications hadn't helped. Finally, Janie's psychologist referred her to us for neurofeedback.

One of the main themes of this book is how emotional pain and physical pain are deeply intertwined. Chronic physical pain can cause us to encapsulate the pain by tensing muscles around it, attempting to hold the pain at bay in narrow focus. Chronic narrow focus can lead to or amplify anxiety, depression, and other emotions. The worse the emotional pain is, the more we tend to narrow-focus and avoid the anxiety and depression. Emotions, as we know, can cause pain that might not be there otherwise. Remember Dr. Lenz's study of neuromodules? Repressed emotion can trigger feelings of pain, via the brain, even if there is nothing detectably wrong in the body.

Other researchers have made related findings. At Northwestern University's Feinberg School of Medicine, a study published in the *Journal of Neuroscience* found that healthy brains maintain a state of equilibrium. When one part of the brain activates, others neutralize. When a person suffers chronic pain, parts of the cortex associated with emotion do not disengage. Dr. Dante Chialvo calls it the brain that "never shuts up." A brain that is constantly running in overdrive sometimes causes permanent damage in connections between brain cells or even death to some brain cells.

Pain exacts other tolls. Another Feinberg School associate professor, A. Vania Apkarian, led a research team that found that brain volume shrinks when chronic pain conditions are present. In a 2004 *Journal of Neuroscience* study, he found that the brains of people in chronic back pain shrink 11 percent—the equivalent of ten to twenty years of normal aging. His earlier research showed that chronic pain also changes brain chemistry and that people with chronic pain take longer to solve crossword puzzles. Clearly, chronic pain must be brought under control to limit such damaging effects.

Another researcher, Stafford Lightman at Bristol University in England, has demonstrated that stress can decrease the quantity of brain cells and cause memory problems. My work suggests that Open Focus can reduce or eliminate stress, preventing such neural damage and loss of function—as well as the physical and emotional pain that often results from chronic stress. By bringing about synchrony and a balance of attention styles, Open-Focus training can quiet overactivity in the brain, counteracting both stress and pain.

Working with Multiple Forms of Pain

In a complicated case like Janie's, with many layers, I try to dissolve one symptom at a time, usually starting with the highest-intensity one. Emotional symptoms such as anxiety and depression are as susceptible to dissolution as physical symptoms, and I started treating Janie by addressing her symptoms of anxiety.

In my view, anxiety and depression are often intertwined. Most of the depression I treat (though not all) is the result of an unconscious attempt to control and reduce feelings of anxiety by reflexively denying, avoiding, or masking feelings of fear in the body. When the anxiety is dissolved, the need to control anxiety by repressing it also disappears and depression can lift on its own, or it can be easily dissolved. In any case, resistance to feelings of depression can be dissolved directly along with the feeling of depression itself. Anxiety can also greatly exacerbate physical pain, making it the logical place to start.

The first order of business in dissolving anxiety is the same as it is with physical pain. I asked Janie to feel the space in the room and maintain this feeling throughout the exercises. The feeling of space starts to wake the body up, allowing the client to become aware of repressed feelings. Then I asked her to locate the most intense feelings of anxiety in her body. At first, many clients say their anxiety is in their mind or all over the body, but anxiety, if we search for it, is usually strongest in one specific location, often the stomach or chest, though it can be anywhere. All anxiety is associated with a feeling in the body, but it's a big step to realize that it's not a general feeling but lives somewhere specific. Sometimes I have clients do a body inventory, asking if the feeling of anxiety is in their toes, feet, ankles, upper legs, and so forth. This exercise continues until the entire body has been surveyed for the sometimes elusive feeling of anxiety and the strongest source or location is discovered.

Sometimes I ask clients to do an inventory with finger pressure, one spot at a time, until they discover where the most pain is generated. Pressing serves as a guide to bring their attention to that spot and allow the pain to diffuse by simply becoming aware of it and immersing into the pain and the space that pervades the pain.

When the clients say they have found it—and they almost always do if they stay with the process of localizing pain—I ask them to feel it more fully and intimately. When Janie located her anxiety in her chest, in the context of space, and began to feel it more fully, I asked her to feel the shape of the space the anxiety occupied. Then she proceeded to dissolve it with Open-Focus dissolving pain techniques.

As a client dissolves high-intensity anxieties, lesser anxieties often release as well. And not infrequently, feelings that don't seem associated with anxiety also disappear, such as muscle tension. However, the first site a client might identify with tension is not always where the most tension or anxiety is. Some people report holding feeling in their jaw, for example. I'll ask them if that's where they feel anxiety, and they'll say yes. More questioning, however, reveals that the anxiety is elsewhere, perhaps in their throat or stomach, and they are tensing their jaw to suppress, mask, or avoid feeling it.

During the first session, Janie self-reported that she was able to reduce her feelings of anxiety by only about 15 percent, which is a comparatively poor result, and almost all of this anxiety returned shortly after the session. It wasn't until the sixth session that Janie was able to dissolve significant amounts of anxiety and physical pain during our office sessions and at home.

Once much of the anxiety has been dissolved, I move on to physical pain. I ask many of my clients to assess their pain on a scale of 0 to 10, with 10 being the most intense, representing a feeling the client can't stand anymore. (This is a standard clinical measure of pain.)

During the sixth session, Janie dissolved chronic upper back and spine pain from 6 to 0, and chronic right shoulder pain from 4 to 0. By the next session, she said she started feeling "happy" for the first time (even before we began dissolving feelings of depression and sadness). By the ninth session—after we had spent two sessions dissolving feelings of depression—she said she felt 100 percent better.

Janie continued to dissolve feelings of depression and sadness, and these were reduced to 0. During the tenth session, she told me that she was once again doing chores around the house. It might not sound like much, but for Janie, as for many of my clients, the ability to do something most of us take for granted is a big victory. Over the course of a few weeks, her life returned to nearly normal.

Most of Janie's physical pain and other symptoms resulting from the accident ameliorated during the period of weeks that we focused on her anxiety and depression. Narrow-objective focus upon the pain, remember, greatly exacerbates the feeling of pain, and changing to diffuse-immersed attention eases even extreme pain. After the anxiety and depression eased, it was easier to access the remaining physical and emotional pain, which included pain in her spine and shoulder blades, a sense of overall heaviness, a broken feeling, numbness, neck and head tension, burning in the upper spine, fear in her heart, anger at the truck driver who fled the scene and left her pinned by the telephone pole, nightmares, waking insomnia, and other fleeting negative emotions. All were mitigated by daily home practice of dissolving pain techniques and office sessions of EEG synchrony training.

Stress, Pain, and the Immune System

There are other ways that our reaction to emotional stress can cause physical pain. Stress has long been shown to have an impact on the immune system; in fact, the field of psychoneuroimmunology (PNI) is devoted solely to understanding the connections between psychological processes and the nervous and immune systems. Because the immune system defends us against so many biological invasions, when the system is compromised by stress, the consequences can be far-reaching. How the stress-impacted immune system causes many types of pain, from headaches to chronic muscle pain to stomach pain, is becoming increasingly studied. One cause is the inflammatory substances that are released in abundance by immune cells when we are under stress, which can contribute to chronic pain.

Immune cells may also cause what is known as neuropathic pain. Pain can be separated into two broad categories: nociceptive and neuropathic. Nociceptive pain is the pain caused by injuries to the body that stimulate pain receptors. Neuropathic pain is created by a malfunction in the nervous system. This type of pain, often chronic, is usually a burning or shooting pain. It's common among patients with cancer and diabetes. Small cells in the nervous system are activated and amplify any existing pain signals.

Immune system–induced pain can assume many forms. Take the case of Kent, who came to see me for severe food allergies. They were so debilitating he needed daily antihistamine injections to keep from throwing up after eating. He could eat only a few plain foods: free-range chicken, organic brown rice, and spinach. Even those caused him to vomit or caused stomach pain after he ate. He suffered chronic low-level headaches as well.

His emotional history was difficult, too. His mother had died when he was a preschooler, and his father was distant, demanding, and prone to anger. In his profession, he drove himself intensely, working full-time and going to night school.

Kent came seeking help for his emotional stress, particularly anger and exhaustion. He didn't expect help with his pain and allergies, he said, because they were not a result of his stress—they were "physical." After a few sessions, though, he noticed that his food reactions did not seem as severe. Then he came for a week-long Open-Focus intensive training seminar. During the sessions, which last for several hours a day, he noticed feelings of fear and anger rise up, and he learned to dissolve them.

Two days into the seminar, Kent was feeling good and de-cided, against my advice, to stop taking his allergy medications. He had no problems, and by the end of the week, he felt as good without the allergy shots as he had while taking them. He also found he could eat a much wider variety of foods without vomit-ing or pain. After several more weeks of home training, he could eat almost anything he chose.

Kent had been tested for allergies before he began Open-Focus training, and when he completed his training, he was tested again. Instead of testing negative, much to my surprise, he still tested positive for the allergies. What had changed, however, was his body's reaction to the allergens.

The stomach and intestines are one of those places in the body where emotional stress and pain are often centered. Researchers believe there is a kind of second brain, something known as the enteric nervous system, in the digestive system (the esophagus, stomach, small intestine, and colon). Surprisingly, there are half a billion neurons in the digestive system—the largest number found outside the central nervous system—as well as neurotransmitters. The enteric system is considered to function as a single, indepen-dent nervous system, with the capacity to learn, remember, and produce what we call gut feelings.

Other Success Stories

Susan Shor Fehmi was treating a sixteen-year-old high-function-ing autistic girl, teaching her how to dissolve pain. This young woman usually played with a doll during sessions, because it helped her feel more comfortable. This time she was playing with her doll, and Susan couldn't get her attention. Exasperated, her father walked across the room, took the doll away, and said a few angry words to the girl. As she got more upset, Susan asked her what she was feeling and where she felt it in her body.

She told Susan that she felt anger, and it was located in her belly. Susan asked her if she could feel the space in the whole room, and the girl said she could. Susan then asked her if she could feel the space her anger occupied, and if she could, what was its size and shape?

"It's like a baseball," she said.

Susan asked her to feel into it, to dissolve it, and she did. This is the heart of the process: Become aware of the feeling, locate it, and dissolve it. With practice, this can all be done reflexively and in short order. We've found that young people can often do it easily and quite quickly.

Stabilizing the brain with flexible attention and ending RAS makes many different systems less reactive and decreases tension throughout the body. People become calmer and less emotionally reactive. It also helps conditions in which the body's muscles seem to take on a life of their own, such as stuttering, tics, Tourette's syndrome, and restless leg syndrome.

I had a client, a young man, who suffered a range of painful tics—head jerks, arching back, involuntary jumping, frequent blinking, and some vocal sounds. People who have these kinds of disorders say that stress exacerbates their problem and that having these kinds of displays causes embarrassment and more stress, as well as muscle tension, which in turn makes their problem worse. This young man tried a host of different doctors and medications before finding a drug called risperidone (or Risperdal), which reduced his tics, but not enough for him.

"When I started Open-Focus training, I felt a difference right away," he wrote me in a letter after his treatment ended. "I had a steady period of feeling good, about two weeks. Since I was feeling better, I started going to school and was enjoying my life better than I had in a long time." He learned how to dissolve anxiety as it rose in him and to feel muscle tension and dissolve that as well. "All of my tics improved. A few of them are still there, but they are not as severe as they used to be (90 percent less). Even though I don't feel 100 percent better, my life has become more enjoyable."

Dissolved symptoms can return depending on how well clients learn to move out—and remain out—of chronic effortful forms of narrow-objective attention and instead adopt a stable Open-Focus attention. How long clients maintain a state of well-being depends on how often they do their Open-Focus exercises and how well they can maintain an Open Focus in daily life. (A later exercise called "Using Open Focus in Daily Life" helps with that.) Depression and anxiety take years to form, under immensely powerful emotional circumstances, and they form in both the brain and the body. If clients habitually return to, and get stuck in, a chronic narrow focus, they can, over time, bring on these unpleasant feelings again.

That's why I encourage people to use these negative feelings as feedback. If they start to feel anxious or depressed, or other unpleasant feelings return, the negative feelings can serve as a reminder to move into Open Focus for symptom dissolution. The pain assumes its appropriate function and becomes feedback, a reminder that it needs to be dissolved. With continued practice, there are longer and longer intervals between recurrences of the pain, until it stops coming back.

One of the most critical lessons informing this book is the integral relationship between physical pain and emotional pain. Most of the clients I've written about experience resolution of physical pain and emotional pain at the same time. The two forms of pain are deeply and inseparably intertwined. Dr. Andrew Weil has written that he has "seen a great many cases of chronic back pain disappear as if by magic when people fall in love or otherwise make radical changes in their emotional and mental life."

There is science to support such ideas. Several researchers at UCLA, in a study published in the journal *Psychological Science* in

November 2009, found that simply looking at a photograph of a loved one can reduce painful feelings. Psychologists studied twenty-five women, mostly students at UCLA who had been in a relationship with a boyfriend for at least six months. While researchers applied moderately painful heat to their forearm, they were shown photographs of an object, a stranger, or their boyfriend. They all reported significantly less pain while looking at the photo of their boyfriend. In another part of the study, the women experienced moderate pain while holding the hand of their boyfriend, a stranger, or holding a ball. All reported less pain while holding their boyfriend's hand.

I deeply believe this is true, for I have seen it here at my clinic as well. Love is very much a way of paying attention. When we are in love, we reduce narrow-objective focus and open up to include more diffuse and immersed styles of attending, which immediately relax the sympathetic nervous system. And these open and immersed styles of attending dissolve the pain.

Can you imagine loving your pain into dissolution?

Exercise

Dissolving Head, Neck, and Shoulder Pain

Take a moment now to adjust your posture so it is gently upright. As best as you can, let yourself be still during the exercise.

Can you imagine letting your mind and body naturally and effortlessly respond to the following questions concerning your ability to imagine certain experiences?

Can you imagine not giving any particular effort to listening to the questions or to achieving any of the associated images or experiences?

Can you imagine that the ideal response is whatever spontaneously happens to your imagery or experience when a particular question is asked? The nature of your experience will naturally change and deepen with continued practice.

Can you imagine that your opening and expanding awareness of your emerging experience is a continuing process?

Can you imagine feeling your most intense pain in your head, neck, or shoulders and rating it on a scale of 0 to 10, with 10 signifying that you can't stand the pain any more, and 0 signifying no pain at all?

Can you imagine feeling the space between your eyes?

Can you imagine feeling the space between your pain and your eyes?

Is it possible for you to imagine feeling the space inside your nose as you inhale and exhale naturally?

Can you imagine feeling your pain and feeling your breath flowing behind and through your eyes as you inhale and exhale naturally?

Can you imagine feeling the space between your pain and the space inside your nose and inside your eyes?

Can you imagine feeling the space inside your throat as you inhale and exhale naturally?

Is it possible for you to imagine feeling the space between your pain and the space inside your throat, and the space inside your nose?

Can you imagine feeling the space between your pain and inside your mouth and cheeks?

Is it possible for you to imagine feeling the space between your pain and the volume of your tongue?

Can you imagine feeling the space between your pain and the volume of your teeth and gums?

Can you imagine feeling the space between your pain and the volume of your lips?

Is it possible for you to imagine feeling the space between your pain and the region between your upper lip and the base of your nose?

Can you imagine feeling the space between your pain and the space inside your throat?

Can you imagine the space between your pain and the inside of your ears?

Can you imagine feeling the space between your pain and the tip of your chin?

Can you imagine the distance between your pain and your temples?

Can you imagine feeling the space between your pain and the top of your head?

Can you imagine feeling the space between your pain and your cheekbones?

Is it possible for you to imagine feeling the space between your pain and the tip of your chin and your eyes?

Can you imagine feeling the space between your pain and the tip of your chin and the middle of your forehead?

Can you imagine feeling the space between your pain and the tip of your chin and the corners of your mouth?

Can you imagine feeling the space between your pain and the tip of your chin and your lower lip?

Is it possible for you to imagine feeling the space between your pain and your whole jaw?

Can you imagine feeling the space between your pain and inside the bridge of your nose?

Can you imagine feeling the space between your pain and the space at the back of your head?

Can you imagine feeling the space between your pain and the space inside your eyes?

Is it possible for you to imagine feeling that the region around your eyes is filled with space?

Can you imagine feeling the space your eyelids occupy?

Can you imagine feeling the space between your pain and your eyelids and your eyebrows?

Is it possible for you to imagine feeling the space between your pain and your entire face simultaneously, including your eyes, ears, forehead, temples, and your jaw and your nose and your tongue, teeth and gums, and lips?

Can you imagine feeling the space between your pain and the region of your scalp?

Can you imagine that as you inhale naturally your breath fills the entire volume of your face and scalp and head including your ears and jaw and eyes?

Can you imagine that as you exhale and as your breath leaves your body it leaves your face, scalp, and head empty, that is, filled with space?

Can you imagine feeling the space between your pain and the space inside your neck and the tips of your shoulders?

Can you imagine feeling the space inside your throat and neck expanding to fill the entire region of your shoulders?

Can you imagine that as you inhale naturally your breath fills your entire head, neck, and shoulders, and that as you exhale and as your breath leaves your body, and it leaves this entire region filled with space?

At the same time you're aware of the space inside this entire region, is it possible for you also to imagine the space around these regions, space around your shoulders and neck and head?

Can you imagine feeling the space the whole room occupies?

Can you imagine also feeling the space your whole body occupies?

Can you imagine also feeling the space your head occupies?

Can you imagine also feeling the space your pain occupies?

Can you imagine letting this awareness, which is you, intermingle with the pain and letting your pain intermingle with your awareness?

Can you imagine letting awareness and pain intermingle, merge, and spread in every direction?

Once again, please rate your remaining pain on a scale of 0 to 10. Can you imagine repeating the preceding six questions until your pain is completely dissolved?

Can you imagine that as you continue to practice, your experience will become more vivid, engaged, and more effortless?

Can you imagine practicing this exercise at least twice daily?

11

Dissolving Tension and Pain
for Peak Performance

Pain is weakness leaving the body.
—Anonymous

A FEW YEARS AGO, John, an investment adviser from New York, became a client. After several sessions, Open Focus "clicked" for John, and it greatly helped to relieve the stress associated with his job. "The first thing I noticed," he said, "was that I was gripping the world around me. My eyes were tired, because I had been straining with my eyes and never realized it. I was astounded to realize the amount of gripping that was taking place, and my hands were often icy cold, which is also part of gripping."

After some Open-Focus sessions, John said his squinting with his brows and eyes dissipated, and his hands warmed up.

One day, well into our sessions, I mentioned I was leaving for Florida the following month, and he lit up. He was going south to play golf at the same time and asked if, while I was there, I could help with a problem he suffered called the yips.

The yips are a movement disorder in sports that is probably best known for its impact on putting in golf. While a golfer prepares to tap the ball gently for a three- or four-foot putt, he or she overswings, often wildly, and the ball goes well beyond the hole. This problem is especially pronounced in older golfers, including the pros, and may, according to one study, afflict as many as half of all golfers.

The term *yips* is credited to Tommy Armour, a golf champion who had to quit playing golf because of them, and they are also known as twitches or jerks. Even the famous Slammin' Sammy Snead came down with the yips, and his putting game was, according to one account, "painful to watch." According to a study by the Mayo Clinic, there are two etiologies, Type I and Type II. Type I is associated with a neurological disorder called dystonia, a kind of cramping in the muscles. Type II is a kind of extreme performance anxiety.

The yips are not only a problem with putting, for they affect full swings and other strokes. And they are not only a problem in golf. Competitors in darts, baseball, cricket, almost any sport, have a version of the yips that interferes with the normal execution of a simple act. There are professional baseball catchers who can no longer throw the ball to second base and professional basketball players who can no longer make a free throw.

In golf, people try to adapt with several strategies. "For years, I had to putt left-handed even though I'm right-handed, or putt split-handed (switching the hand position on the club), but nothing seemed to work," John said. "I read books, tried ten different putters, went to a golf clinic, but nothing helped. Every other part of my game was fine, except for putting. I'd line up the ball and start to putt, but in the process of stroking, my muscles in my wrists and forearms twitch, almost like a miniseizure. The ball goes zooming off in any direction, and it causes enormous amounts of doubt and anxiety. There's some malfunction, a movement that you cannot control. I'm an excellent golfer, but when the yips came, I gave up the game. It was too frustrating and embarrassing, and it seemed unfixable."

I met John in Florida and went with him to a putting green and watched while he putted. As he did, I coached him in becoming aware of space around him and entering into and maintaining an Open Focus. He was already familiar with the feel of Open Focus but needed some instruction on bringing it into play while putting.

"At the end of the session, I experienced a transformation in my putting," says John. "I sank fifteen balls in a row from three feet out. It didn't get completely better that day, but it showed I can do it." He has since done more Open Focus and is playing competitive golf again. "I've returned to putting right-handed, and my game has never been better. I am putting 100 percent with the standard style of putting."

John describes Open Focus as "a general relaxation of the entire system." He continues, "It leads to better movement. I didn't just fix a swing with Open Focus, but I changed my whole game— both golf and tennis. I've never played either so well."

One of the enemies of a smooth and fluid performance, whether in sports, the performing arts, or at work, is pain and tension that keep the body from performing at its best. It's easier to see why pain can hamper performance, but it's a little more difficult to realize that tension—the precursor to pain—is causing the blockage. Often we aren't even aware of the tension that is blocking our performance because we've lived with it so long we no longer realize it's there. John said he didn't feel any tension, but I believe some tension was present nonetheless. And if he had gone deeper with the training, he would probably have found a great deal of tension under the surface.

I've had clients come into the office after having successfully dissolved one or a number of chronic pains and say, "I am good. Everything's good today. There's no pain or emotion that I need to get rid of." I'll ask them to review the last few weeks or months or any time in their history and come up with an event that was accompanied by pain, tension, or other untoward feeling or emotion. Can you think of one? Usually people can. I ask them to visualize and feel the event and then feel the pain, tension, and anxiety that are associated with the experience. I ask them to hold that feeling and visual image in their mind and feel into their body and notice where it is in their body and then proceed to dissolve that pain.

After dissolving previously hidden pain in this way, people actually feel very much better. They get that feeling of lightness and brightness that comes after release, and their performance—athletic or otherwise—is often improved.

Open-Focus training is well suited to golf or any other sport in which different styles of attention are used for different parts of the game. Fifteen or twenty minutes of Open-Focus exercise before a round of golf loosens muscles and reduces tension. But a good golfer must be able to shift easily among different modes of attention. Placing the ball on the tee and getting ready for a drive call for narrow focus, with its ability to plan a strategy and assess the placement of the tee, the direction of the wind, the location of trees, the distance from other golfers, and so forth. Then, shifting into diffuse attention helps integrate this information and loosen the muscles. Moving into Open Focus at the setup and for the backswing immediately relaxes major muscle groups and facilitates a full and fluid downswing.

A golfer who stays in narrow focus has a one-pointed attention placed almost entirely on the ball. By contrast, in Open Focus, the player gently centers his attention on the ball but simultaneously also includes an awareness of things in the periphery of attention, such as the grass, trees, and other features of the landscape, and, of course, space. During the swing, the golfer's awareness merges into an even fuller experience of oneness with the ball—while still maintaining the center of attention on the ball—to the point that some report their sense of self disappears.

In a study of archers at Arizona State University, Dr. Daniel M. Landers monitored athletes' brain-wave activity with an EEG. He found that when top archers are mentally preparing to shoot, the brain is chattering away at between 13 and 30 hertz—the beta range, characteristic of narrow focus. After the bow is drawn back and the archer is preparing to release it, his or her brain-wave frequency drops into alpha, 8 to 12 hertz, a more open style of attending that calms the brain and body, stops the mental chatter, and allows a fluid dedication and immersion in the task. Numerous studies show that the EEG pattern is the same for rifle shooting, basketball, karate, and pistol shooting.

Often a diffuse focus by itself is enough to dissolve the tension that affects performance. Although Pablo Casals, the virtuoso cellist, in his later years could barely walk without assistance to the chair onstage and prop his instrument between his legs, but when he began to play, he played with vigor and grace. Why? Because through years of practice he instinctively knew how to attend effortlessly while he played. Good flexible attention skills are one of those things that separates a good performer from a great one.

Other times the tension in the hands and arms can be so great that dissolving pain exercises are needed.

During artistic or athletic performance, muscles are almost never completely at rest—they maintain a baseline tension to preserve structural alignment, posture, and balance. This tension or tonus needs to be kept to a minimum, though, so the workload can be distributed in a flexible and coordinated way throughout the body.

I've worked with a number of singers and public speakers whose levels of tension impaired their performance. Open Focus works well for releasing tension in the groin, diaphragm, throat, eyes, and the facial mask. These are all areas where we hold extra tension from emotional stress as we face the world. "All of my singers have this gripping and tension in their facial mask, and they have to let it go," says Rae Tattenbaum, a teacher at the Hartt School of Music in Connecticut. "Once they use Open Focus to release their face muscles, their whole physiology responds and releases. They can better employ the diaphragm. They feel like they own their space onstage, and they can use their performance muscles the way they were meant to be used."

Breaking the grip of rigid attention syndrome, or RAS, and adopting a flexible approach to attention is a sine qua non not only for peak performance in arts and athletics but also for productivity and excellence at work. Take the case of Edward, a stock trader, who came to the clinic complaining of a surprisingly large number of stress-related symptoms, most prominently, gastrointestinal symptoms associated with irritable bowel syndrome, mild headaches, and sleeplessness. Irritable bowel syndrome is often caused by stress, and Edward's job compounded the stress he carried with him from childhood. The IBS was very painful for him, with chronic and often severe abdominal pains, bloating, and alternating diarrhea and constipation. Edward's symptoms reached the point where they were a significant distraction at work.

Many employers understand that pain and tension, part and parcel of on-the-job stress, can make it difficult for employees to concentrate at work. Employers in this country lose more than $60 billion a year to absenteeism and diminished productivity from chronic pain, according to the American Academy of Pain Management.

Like our other clients, Edward was placed on a schedule of Open-Focus home practice and went through several sessions in our clinic. In a few weeks, his pain was gone, he told me, and whenever he was under a great deal of stress, as he had been during recent periods of market volatility, he could return to more restful styles of attention and dissolve his pain. "It was a godsend," he said. For the past five years, he has been the only trader in his company to consistently show a profit.

Many high-functioning people have been taught to think that success depends on pushing harder—and if that doesn't work, then push harder still. It's an idea that is deeply ingrained in our culture. But that is simply not always the case. There are times to narrow focus, and there are times when it is important to adopt other styles of attention. Blending styles of attention appropriately is much more effective than always being in high-speed, narrow-objective focus.

Exercise

Using Open Focus in Daily Life

This exercise is best used after some facility is gained with Open Focus. It reminds and encourages us to bring Open-Focus attention into daily life.

Remember to allow fifteen seconds between the end of one question and the beginning of the next question.

Guiding Questions

Can you imagine what it would be like if you were already successfully resting in Open Focus in this moment?

Can you imagine paying attention to the presence of all senses, attending equally and simultaneously to the objects of sensation and to the space in which sensations occur?

Can you imagine a narrow-absorbed attention surrounded by a diffuse-objective attention?

Can you imagine in detail the following activities, as you experience them in Open Focus?

Can you imagine paying attention in Open Focus while anticipating your day, your week, your month, your lifetime?

Can you imagine paying attention in Open Focus while awakening in the morning?

Can you imagine attending in Open Focus while dressing and preparing yourself for the day?

Can you imagine paying attention in Open Focus while eating breakfast?

Can you imagine attending in Open Focus while commuting?

Can you imagine paying attention in Open Focus during meetings?

Can you imagine attending in Open Focus during breaks?

Can you imagine paying attention in Open Focus during lunch?

Can you imagine attending in Open Focus while thinking?

Can you imagine attending in Open Focus while writing?

Can you imagine paying attention in Open Focus while answering the phone?

Can you imagine attending in Open Focus while setting priorities?

Can you imagine paying attention in Open Focus while listening to music or other sounds?

Can you imagine attending in Open Focus while socializing?

Can you imagine paying attention in Open Focus while answering questions?

Can you imagine attending in Open Focus while watching TV, a play, or a movie?

Can you imagine attending in Open Focus during interruptions?

Can you imagine attending in Open Focus while being evaluated?

Can you imagine attending in Open Focus while receiving criticism?

Can you imagine paying attention in Open Focus while cleaning and organizing?

Can you imagine attending in Open Focus while receiving praise?

Can you imagine paying attention in Open Focus while exercising and playing sports?

Can you imagine paying attention in Open Focus while doing work you dislike?

Can you imagine paying attention in Open Focus while engaging in physical labor?

Can you imagine attending in Open Focus while responding to a deadline?

Can you imagine paying attention in Open Focus while paying bills?

Can you imagine attending in Open Focus while dealing with people you don't like?

Can you imagine attending in Open Focus while feeling emotional?

Can you imagine attending in Open Focus to a task you would like to avoid today?

Can you imagine paying attention in Open Focus while speaking with your parents?

Can you imagine paying attention in Open Focus while speaking with your children?

Can you imagine attending in Open Focus while doing something pleasurable or exciting?

Can you imagine paying attention in Open Focus while arguing with someone?

Can you imagine paying attention in Open Focus while responding to an emergency?

Can you imagine attending in Open Focus while shopping?

Can you imagine paying attention in Open Focus while driving?

Can you imagine attending in Open Focus while preparing meals?

Can you imagine paying attention in Open Focus while daydreaming?

Can you imagine paying attention in Open Focus while worrying?

Can you imagine paying attention in Open Focus while waiting?

Can you imagine attending in Open Focus during dinner?

Can you imagine paying attention in Open Focus while feeling stressed?

Can you imagine paying attention in Open Focus during leisure time?

Can you imagine paying attention in Open Focus while playing games?

Can you imagine attending in Open Focus while pursuing meaningful relationships?

Can you imagine paying attention in Open Focus during intimate moments?

Can you imagine attending in Open Focus while preparing for bed?

Can you imagine attending in Open Focus while reading?

Can you imagine paying attention in Open Focus while falling asleep?

Can you imagine attending in Open Focus while sleeping and dreaming?

Can you imagine attending in Open Focus while practicing Open-Focus exercises?

Can you imagine attending in Open Focus while feeling body tension?

Can you imagine attending in Open Focus while feeling the discomfort of self-consciousness?

Can you imagine attending in Open Focus while feeling the pangs of hunger?

Can you imagine attending in Open Focus while feeling physical pain?

Can you imagine this is the end of this exercise and the beginning of Open Focus for the rest of your life?

12

Living a Pain-Free Life

*We have not been informed that our bodies do what they
are told, if we know how to tell them.*

—ELMER GREEN, BIOFEEDBACK PIONEER

IMAGINE OWNING a sports car, an expensive, exquisitely designed piece of equipment that superbly handles all kinds of driving conditions. Imagine, though, that you were never taught to drive properly and for years you drove the car in just two gears. Something seemed not quite right, but you got used to it, and after a while it seemed fine. Then one day a friend comes by and says, "Can I drive it?"

"Sure," you say, and you get in next to him and head out on a winding road, where the friend, who knows how to drive, expertly shifts between all six gears.

"Holy cow," you think to yourself. "I've been driving this thing wrong all this time. It is a much more high-performance machine than I ever imagined."

So it is with the human central nervous system. Chronic pain is largely the product of not knowing how to properly operate the mind-body system. We have control over aspects of our physiology that seem beyond our control. It's been well researched and established, but somehow forgotten.

In addition to the research presented earlier, in the 1960s, John Basmajian, a Canadian researcher, was studying motor units, an organized pathway of nerve cells that extends from the brain down the spine and out to the muscles. He placed a tiny needle electrode into the muscle at the base of the thumb and amplified the sound of a firing neuron making clicks on a small speaker. Eight of Basmajian's sixteen subjects were able to learn to fire those few cells at will and make clicking sounds on the speaker. After a little bit of practice, the subjects learned to play distinctive rhythms by firing these cells. They could imitate the sound of a horse galloping or do drumrolls when asked. They didn't know how they could do it, they said, they just could.

Basmajian's work, which he wrote about in his 1979 book *Muscles Alive,* astounded the nascent field of the operant conditioning of autonomic responses, which later became known as biofeedback. Do we really have that level of control over our physiology?

The answer is yes, and Open-Focus attention training is about learning how to control functions that seem beyond control and putting this ability to work effortlessly to reduce or eliminate pain, among other applications.

The first big breakthrough in the field came in the late 1950s. Neal E. Miller, doing research at Yale, proved he could teach lab animals to alter certain autonomic functions, at the time considered independent of voluntary control.

Miller investigated rats to see if they could control their heartbeat. To eliminate the possibility they were using the muscles in their chest, he injected them with curare, used by tribes in South America to paralyze their prey. He stuck an electrode into the pleasure center of the rats' brains, and every time they lowered or raised their heart rate, he gave them a jolt of good feeling. Within ninety minutes, they were able to alter their heart rate upon command by 20 percent.

Miller then moved on to human subjects, a group of patients with an abnormally fast heartbeat. Whenever a subject's heart rate fell to a healthy level, he was rewarded with a pleasant tone. And he taught subjects at Harvard Medical School to raise and lower their blood pressure. (Incidentally, the subjects in this study were males, and their reward, when they changed their blood pressure in the desired way, was a glance at a *Playboy* centerfold— not exactly the type of feedback one would see in such studies today.)

Some of the early operant-conditioning research that gained a great deal of attention was the operant conditioning of brain waves. As I mentioned earlier, the first to realize we could control our brain waves was Dr. Joe Kamiya, a researcher at the Langley Porter Neuropsychiatric Institute. He designed an experiment to see if the subjects could tell what frequency range their brains were in.

During the first session of the first experiment, the subject seemed to be guessing what frequency range he was experiencing. But by the third and fourth sessions, the first subject could easily tell when he was in alpha. By the fourth session, the young man correctly guessed his brain state *four hundred times in a row*. Kamiya was astounded that this subject could so successfully recognize his own EEG activity.

In follow-up experiments, Kamiya wanted to see if the student could generate alpha at will. "Go into the alpha state when you hear a bell ring once," the young man was told. "If it rings twice, do not go into alpha." The student was able to control his brain waves perfectly. Others also learned control of their brain waves.

What captured the imagination of the public, though, was the fact that people who learned to generate alpha at will left the experiments feeling calm, clear, and refreshed. It was the first modern alpha training, and it led to the field of neurofeedback, teaching people to handle many stress-related problems on their own. There has been a rebirth of brain-wave training around the world, with thousands of practitioners using neurofeedback to treat attention deficit disorder, hyperactivity, anxiety, chronic pain, and a host of other disorders.

Elmer and Alyce Green of the Menninger Clinic also studied the phenomenon of self-regulation. The Greens took a portable research lab to India to study Eastern holy men. The subject of one of the most intriguing experiments was Yogiraja Vaidyaraja, the so-called burying yogi, who often spent two or three days buried in a box several feet underground to demonstrate his spiritual development and devotion.

For the purposes of the test, Yogiraja Vaidyaraja was seated in the lotus position in a completely airtight wooden cube measuring three and a half feet by three and a half feet by five feet. One panel of the crate was a door, made of quarter-inch plate glass, through which the Greens and their team could see the yogi. The cracks around the door were sealed with a quarter inch of foam. Green felt the box was sealed more tightly than a refrigerator. An associate of the yogi burned a candle in the box, and it went out, for lack of oxygen, after ninety minutes.

Instruments were attached to the yogi to measure, among other things, his heart rate, his galvanic skin response (GSR), which measures the rate of sweating, and his EEG. The Greens thought the yogi would reach his limit in two hours, while a doctor present said he would need to be let out after four hours to avoid losing consciousness.

After nearly eight hours in the airless box, the yogi signaled to the researchers that he wanted to be let out, complaining that he had received electric shocks from the equipment. Green was astounded. During the yogi's stay in the box, his respiration rate had dropped to less than four breaths per minute, and his pulse rate had dropped by more than half. After the yogi emerged from the box, researchers tried to take a blood sample, and they couldn't—the holy man had stopped the flow of blood to his extremities.

The EEG showed that the yogi "produced alpha almost continuously," the Greens wrote. They also found the yogi had the unusual ability to move quickly between disparate brain frequencies. When he entered the box, he switched nimbly and almost instantly from beta, or normal waking consciousness, into a deep alpha state.

Such experiments are more than just interesting stories—they demonstrate beyond doubt that humans have the power to self-regulate, to control functions we have been led to believe we have no control over.

The goal of Open-Focus training is to gain a measure of voluntary control over our attention and subsequently over our physiology in order to manage pain. While it may take years for someone to become as adept as the burying yogi, learning to control attention styles, and managing our pain, can be accomplished in fairly short order.

Step by step, the Open-Focus exercises teach us to move effortlessly out of narrow-objective focus into a more open, immersed style of attending. This in itself often releases accumulated stress and tension and allows us to feel better, lighter, clearer, and more present in the now. Eventually, we can move awareness closer to our pain to dissolve it. Other exercises teach us to maintain this awareness on a daily basis. These exercises are pieces of a whole, learned one at a time. It's similar to learning to play the guitar: first we learn to hold the instrument, then we learn to find the notes on the neck, and then how to strum the strings. Then we learn to put these skills together to play a song.

With practice, we can learn to move into Open Focus seamlessly, as second nature, using our ability to attend flexibly. That means dissolving pain and tension as they begin to form in our awareness. When we learn to dissolve pain, the pain becomes an important signal, a prompt to shift attention styles. The idea is to catch pain as it arises, before it becomes monumental and permanent, to merge with the pain and truly dissolve it, as opposed to distracting ourselves from it as most of us normally do.

Integral to Open-Focus training is developing our awareness of space. Becoming aware of space helps keep us from getting stuck in narrow-objective focus. To optimize our mental and physical health, we need to apportion as much attentional importance to space as we do to objects, feelings, and thoughts.

We can meet much of life's pain with these skills and not only dissolve pain but get more out of life, and make it a much deeper and richer experience. Over the years, two clients who had learned to dissolve their anxiety later became pregnant, and both used dissolving pain techniques to merge with and dissolve their childbirth pains. They found their experience at the time of birth to be not only much less painful but much more loving as well. Both were second-time moms and felt they had a better emotional connection at birth with their second child.

A masseuse familiar with Open Focus uses it to teach her clients to dissolve muscle tension while she works on them with her hands. Imagine the space around the tension, she instructs them.

Once dissolving pain skills are learned, you can feel into places where you normally don't experience pain, find hidden tension, and dissolve it as a preventative measure. Remember that tension is a precursor to pain and takes a toll on performance. Many people have said that they didn't know they had pain until they began doing the Open-Focus exercises. Obviously, it was blocked from awareness, and blocking discomfort takes an increasing toll on the body and on performance. As confidence in your ability to dissolve pain grows, it becomes possible to intentionally bring hidden pain to the fore, to let it rise in consciousness so it can be dissolved. By imagining painful situations from the past, we can also acknowledge any associated emotional pain that may have been suppressed and dissolve it using Open Focus—before this blocked emotional tension leads to RAS and physical pain.

There is more recent research that supports the validity of the operant-conditioning model. At the Stanford Systems Neuroscience and Pain Lab, researchers are using functional magnetic resonance imaging, or fMRI, to allow chronic pain patients to see the brain activity associated with their physical pain as it occurs in real time, and to help these patients to learn in short order to reduce that activity and end the pain. It's cutting-edge neurofeedback, the most powerful of all because it allows users to see an image of their brain in operation.

"Everyone is born with a system designed to turn off pain," said Christopher deCharms, a pain researcher with a company called Omneuron, who is working on the fMRI project. "There isn't an obvious mechanism to turn off other diseases like Parkinson's. With pain, the system is there, but most of us haven't initiated control over the intensity dial."

My work indicates that we do in fact have control over the dial—we can control it with our attention. While using modern imaging technology may be a powerful way to turn off pain, so is understanding and gaining control over our ability to direct our attention. It's far less expensive and far more empowering.

Children, incidentally, are very adept learners when it comes to the dissolution of pain. I have taught children in less than five minutes how to feel and dissolve everything from stomachaches to headaches to muscle pain. They are naturally more flexible when it comes to attention and haven't learned all the bad habits of chronic narrow focus. Since children already have flexible attention skills, it would make great sense to teach them to stay flexible with a series of simple exercises that could be integrated into school curricula.

Open-Focus training is available to everyone, to enable them to stop pain and gain control over their lives. It's simple and easy to learn.

Can you imagine a world where you are free from the constant throb, ache, or stabbing of pain and instead live in the broad surround of open awareness and flexible attention?

Many native cultures understood how to dissolve fear, pain, and discomfort. Indigenous peoples had no advanced medical procedures, hospitals, or antidepressants. Young people were schooled in how to manage pain. Coming-of-age rituals were often lessons in learning to dissolve pain—for example, by handling a hot rock. Perhaps these were key opportunities to learn the principle of merging with pain instead of running from it. In our modern culture, we seem to have lost this knowledge of how to self-regulate in response to pain.

In *The Open-Focus Brain,* I wrote about a psychologist friend of mine who went with a medicine man into a Native American sweat lodge, which is something like a smoke-filled sauna. The intense heat and smoke overwhelmed him, and his throat and sinuses burned in pain. But my friend was able to draw on his Open-Focus training and decided to melt into and merge with his discomfort. When he did this, he found that almost instantaneously the pain vanished.

Then something even more remarkable occurred. Reaching into the pile of heated rocks in the center of the lodge, the medicine man picked up a large, very hot stone and handed it to my friend. Again, his Open-Focus training came into play, and he was actually able to melt into and dissolve the pain of holding the stone. The burning sensation stopped, and he was able to hold the rock for a while. Surprised at my friend's ability to manage pain, the medicine man asked him, "Where did you learn to do that?"

Becoming aware of how we attend to our internal and external worlds is, I believe, an emerging aspect of human evolution. What we pay attention to, and how we pay attention to it, dictates our reality. Part of that is the ability to generate an awareness of yourself that is free of pain.

The first step is to understand that we have a range of attention styles to choose from. Then we can move to expand our awareness beyond a narrow scope of attention to a broader aperture, one that admits all peripheral experience at the same time. When we are able to do that, we have expanded our consciousness to the point where we are no longer caught up in, nor overreactive to troublesome stimuli, such as pain, because they are now only a small part of our awareness.

When we fully develop flexible attention skills, we become better adapted to our world—we can be an inclusive, loving being one instant (in diffuse-immersed attention) and an ambitious lawyer devising a strategy for a court appearance (in narrow-objective attention) the next. We can lay down our problems and responsibilities and our pain as we choose and, if appropriate, pick them up again. We can diffuse pain, depression, and anxiety. We can move through life using our attention skills the way they were meant to be used, to have a fuller, richer life, free of pain, anxiety, and worry, one in which we are deeply connected to the people we love. One could say that fully flexible attention gives us the keys to the kingdom.

Exercise

Dissolving Pain (Short Form)

I went to see my optometrist one day, and, after a few pleasantries, I realized he was upset. He told me that he was overcome by grief over his mother's recent death and broke down crying. Knowing that I am a psychologist, he asked me if there was anything that he could do to stop his embarrassing bouts of crying. I offered to teach him Open Focus to manage this crisis, and he was willing to try it. I asked him to feel the space in the whole room and beyond whenever he felt as if he was beginning to be overcome by his grief and crying.

The next time I came to see him, he was beaming. He said being able to feel the space in the whole room, and beyond, helped him greatly. When he did this, he could feel the tension in his chest melting. This is an example of how, with practice, we can quickly dissolve pain.

The following exercise is an abbreviated form of the "Dissolving Pain" exercise presented earlier in the book. Use this exercise, for example, after you've been successfully practicing Open Focus for a period of time. Then the short form can be used when you don't have time for the longer form.

Remember to allow fifteen seconds between the end of one question and the beginning of the next question.

Guiding Questions

Can you imagine paying attention to any feeling of chronic pain that is present right now? (Keep in mind that if you don't feel a well-defined pain, you can address any unpleasant sensation, such as chronic tension, pressure, weakness, tingling, or heaviness.)

Can you localize your pain? Can you imagine feeling where in your body your pain is most intense?

Is it in your throat, chest, stomach, or perhaps behind your eyes? It can be anywhere in your body, around your body, or in your mind.

If you have found 100 percent of your strongest chronic pain in a particular location in your body, choose a number on a 0 to 10 scale, which represents the intensity of this pain.

If you have localized less than 100 percent of your strongest pain, imagine what percentage remains unlocalized, and repeat the process of localization until all the pain has been found at one or more particular locations in your body.

Can you imagine paying attention to the feeling of space in the whole room you are in?

Can you imagine paying attention to the feeling of space your body occupies?

Can you imagine paying attention to the feeling of space your pain occupies?

Can you imagine gently placing your attention underneath the location of the pain and, in slow motion, floating upward, until you arrive at the heart-center of your pain?

Can you imagine the pain spreading through this attention, which is you, through your body, through the boundaries of your body, through the space your body occupies, and through the space in the room in every direction, simultaneously?

Can you imagine experiencing immersed attention, that is, a feeling of absorption, when you feel the pain spreading?

Can you now imagine rating on a 0 to 10 scale the intensity of the remaining pain?

Can you imagine repeating the cycle of objectifying and merging with your pain, then using a 0 to 10 scale to rate the intensity of remaining pain?

Can you imagine repeating these questions, moving toward any remaining pain from various directions? For example, can you imagine letting this immersed attention, which is you, float down into the pain from above, or letting it float from in front of the pain, or from behind, or from the sides, into the center of the feeling of pain?

Can you imagine repeating this process until the pain is completely dissolved?

Can you imagine dissolving the next most intense remaining pain? First by localizing, in the body, the most intense physical or emotional pain. Second, by letting that awareness, which is you, merge with your pain, letting your pain spread through the surrounding body and space. Third, by paying objective attention again to how much pain remains and rating the intensity of the remaining pain on a 0 to 10 scale.

Can you imagine again merging with any remaining pain and letting the pain spread in any direction?

Creating a Personal Program
for Dissolving Pain

Wisdom is nothing more than healed pain.
—Robert Gary Lee, author and actor

This appendix offers guidance on how to use the Open-Focus techniques and exercises in an ongoing way to manage chronic pain and stress in your own life.

First, it's important to realize that you can practice the simple techniques of Open Focus anywhere—on the subway, in your living room, in the yard raking leaves, in the office—simply by opening your awareness to the experience of space. In your daily life, let any unpleasant sensations that may arise become your reminders, your signals, to shift your awareness to space. Becoming aware of space, feeling the space in and around you, for even a few seconds can lead to a release of pain and stress. The longer you maintain an awareness of space, the deeper the release.

Yet it can be hard for most of us to maintain an awareness of space on our own for more than a few minutes. So the Open-Focus exercises are designed to offer a twenty- or thirty-minute experience of space. In preparation for listening to an Open-Focus exercise, find a quiet spot. I recommend that people sit upright in a chair, if possible. Some people lie on a bed, but that can lead to sleep. Falling asleep is not wrong or a bad thing, but we get more out of an exercise if we stay awake. Many people tell me that doing an exercise first thing in the morning is most effective. Try not to practice after a large meal, which can make you more sleepy. There are wide variations in response to the Open-Focus exercises. None of them are wrong, so stay with the practices, even if you feel unsure or uncomfortable. The key to using these exercises is to develop a sense of effortlessness, of allowing your experience to unfold, rather than a sense of effortful trying. If you have difficulty imagining any particular experience or image, don't let that trouble you. If you find your mind wanders or is focused on some thought or image, neither resist nor encourage this.

As you do an exercise, you may notice shooting pains, jerks, tremors, twitches, numbness or tingling feelings, fatigue, anxiety, perspiration, thoughts, memories, or feelings that spontaneously rise into consciousness. If this happens, simply witness it without judgment, including it in your Open-Focus awareness. You may also experience spontaneous pleasant sensations, such as a warming of your feet, a release of head and body tension, clarity, peacefulness, and well-being.

The Progression of Exercises

Begin with "General Training in Open Focus" (track 2 of the audio CD), which takes you through an awareness of space throughout your body. Listen to this exercise for a week or so at least twice a day. This will release some tension and stress, and perhaps some pain, and provide a feeling of Open Focus.

If your pain doesn't resolve by doing the general training exercise, begin working with the "Dissolving Pain" exercise (track

3). If the dissolving pain exercise doesn't bring about a favorable result then try the localization of pain exercise. When the pain is fully localized then try the dissolving pain exercise again. In any case use the general training and dissolving pain exercises until you are successful, or until you give up temporarily. Can you imagine revisiting these exercises from time to time for further gain?

Let's say you have chronic lower back pain, one of the most common complaints. The "Dissolving Pain" exercise takes you on a tour through your whole body and asks you to feel the space between the back pain and different parts of your body. This allows a larger awareness to form around the pain, and because the pain has been placed within the context of this bigger space, you are no longer afraid of being overwhelmed by the pain. The exercise ends with a merging of awareness into the heart of the localized pain, which allows it to diffuse throughout your whole body and into surrounding space. Use the "Dissolving Pain" exercise for a week, two or three times a day.

In the hands of a certified Open Focus trainer most people dissolve their initial presenting pain in one session. Our feeling here at the Princeton Biofeedback Centre is that the least expensive, least invasive, and safest approaches should be tried first, that is, after ruling out the need for other procedures by an appropriate health-care provider.

When you have the time and feel comfortable practicing for longer periods, you will get more benefit using the long form practice. When you don't have enough time, use the short form.

After practicing the General Training in Open Focus exercise for a few weeks, one may notice that pain is experienced less frequently and less intensely, that is even before starting to use the Dissolving Pain exercise. This is because as you begin to open and diffuse attention, stress and pain are diffused also.

It is the intent of this book to empower you to know how to dissolve the pain that negatively affects your quality of life. To live pain-free is a gift. However, my greater hope is that by successfully learning to dissolve your pain, you will also learn how to live in Open-Focus attention and discover that life can be bright, light, and effortless, as well as free of pain. That is an even greater gift.

Index

About the Authors

LES FEHMI, PhD, is director of the Princeton Biofeedback Centre in Princeton, New Jersey. Since the late 1960s, he has been one of the pioneers in the field of bio- and neurofeedback.

For over four decades, Les Fehmi has been active as a psychologist in private practice, a speaker, a biofeedback trainer, and a consultant for such organizations as Harvard Medical School, Johnson & Johnson, the Department of Veterans Affairs, the Dallas Cowboys, and the New Jersey Nets. He holds an MA and a PhD from UCLA. He is the coauthor of *The Open-Focus Brain: Harnessing the Power of Attention to Heal Mind and Body*.

For more information on Dr. Les Fehmi and Open-Focus training, or to order a complete set of Open-Focus exercises on audio CD, visit www.openfocus.com.

JIM ROBBINS is an award-winning journalist and science writer, with frequent contributions to the *New York Times, Smithsonian, Scientific American, Discover,* and *Psychology Today*. He is the author of *A Symphony in the Brain: The Evolution of the New Brain Wave Biofeedback* and coauthor of *The Open-Focus Brain*.

List of Audio Tracks

1. Introduction (15:34)
2. General Training in Open-Focus (28:12)
3. Dissolving Pain with Open Focus (21:27)

The enclosed audio CD includes two essential Open-Focus exercises for dissolving pain that are described in this book. For audio recordings of other exercises, visit openfocus.com.

You can also download the tracks listed above at www .shambhala.com/DissolvingPain.